# The Parkinson's Disease Survival Guide

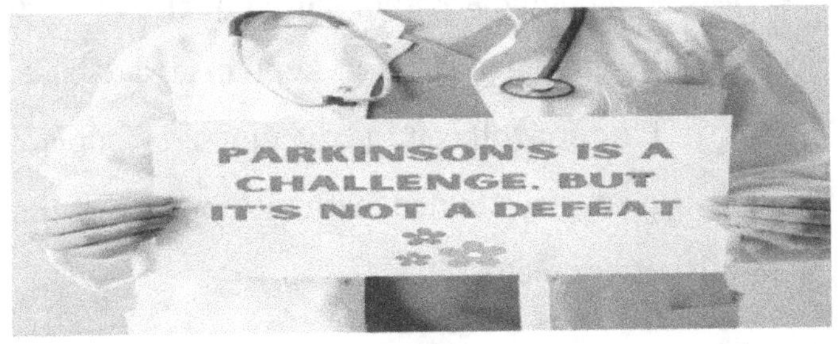


## A Guide for Newly Diagnosed Patients and Their Families

*Dr. Stacia J. Moran*

Copyright © by Dr. Stacia J. Moran 2023. All rights reserved.

Before this document is duplicated or reproduced in any manner, the publisher's consent must be gained. Therefore, the contents within can neither be stored electronically, transferred, nor kept in a database. Neither in Part nor full can the document be copied, scanned, faxed, or retained without approval from the publisher or creator.

# Table of contents

# Introduction

**What Parkinson's Disease Feels Like**

Tremor is one of Parkinson's disease's more widely recognized symptoms. But as time has gone on, we've come to realize that managing movement is just a small part of living with the neurological illness. Everything that the illness can affect, including mental health, memory, energy levels, and more. It can seem absorbing in nature.

Olivia Jackson, a 66-year-old former underground silver miner who now works in sales, says that Parkinson's disease may be frightening and traumatizing. She was given the diagnosis in 2014. You can, however, nonetheless lead a happy life despite this disability.

As she shares how Parkinson's has affected her life, you may learn how this is possible.

**60-year-old Olivia Jackson from Stephens City, Virginia**

I simply could not lift my legs.

By the time Olivia  Jackson saw the doctor for the examination that resulted in a Parkinson's diagnosis, she had been experiencing new symptoms steadily for nearly a year. Before the tremor on her left side, there was the soreness and stiffness in her left shoulder and hand.

She eventually realized she couldn't hang her garments up. A cashier would give Jackson her change, but she couldn't manage to put it in her wallet. She also started experiencing issues with coinage. Her daughter in Northern Ireland also informed her that her phone was moving during video calls.

Jackson remembers that as she moved around, "everything was very intentional." I moved very carefully and deliberately.

Nevertheless, she claims that "Parkinson's was never on the radar for me." However, she started to worry about her mobility one day. After 35 years working in the healthcare industry, she was used to using the stairs rather than the elevator to the fourth floor, so this felt strange to her.

"I noticed that I just could not get my legs lifted," she claims. "I felt as though my capacity to move fast or run down the stairs was fading away. And I reasoned, "You know, I don't know that I would make it out of this building if there were to be a fire." It was very challenging to descend the steps.

When she finally received a diagnosis, she was not only taken aback but also unprepared. Jackson was given a prescription and instructed to schedule a follow-up appointment in six months. That's all there was.

Because we lacked knowledge and were unsure of what this diagnosis indicated, she says, "It was frightening." In some ways, I believe that accepting the diagnosis was easier for me than watching your children and husband struggle with it.

Because you contrast your expectations for your life with what you're actually left with, she claims that you genuinely go through a grieving process. After grieving for a few months, she realized that "my tale isn't going to end here. I still have a lot to do," she declares.

She continues, "I believe it's imperative for people to have purpose in their lives. "I believe that is what separates successful people from unsuccessful people."

It might be challenging for those who have a chronic, disabling neurological ailment like Parkinson's disease to perceive the positive aspects of adversity. Your senses could be clouded by anger, self-pity, and fear. You can become so terrified that you give up. You could experience moments of feeling like a victim, dependent on others to complete even the most basic chores.

There's a chance. Parkinson's disease treatment is advancing thanks to new drugs, operations, a thriving research community, healthcare facilities, and support systems. We might one day even have a treatment.

Today, PD patients have a far better prognosis than they did even ten years ago. New drugs are currently being created. There are services available to simplify your life and the duties of your caretakers. This book will provide you a better understanding of Parkinson's disease, its various therapies, helpful self-help techniques to feel better and stay active, and the numerous benefits of keeping a positive mindset.

What is within of you is far more important than what is in front of you or behind you.

# Chapter one

# Parkinson's Disease Self-Help Techniques

It is simple to feel helpless or think there is nothing you can do if Parkinson's disease (PD) has been diagnosed in you or someone you care about. All in all, PD is a chronic, developing condition for which there is now no treatment. However, there are many things you can do to enhance your life or the life of someone you care about.

Self-help techniques can help people with PD live better lives. Self-help techniques can lessen the severity of symptoms but they cannot reverse the disease. New medications can also stop many severe symptoms from occurring and reduce the progression of the condition. You may keep your freedom for as long as possible by using the self-help methods provided here. Perhaps most significantly, they can improve your sense of peace and tranquility.

# How Can I Help Myself?

Self-help is a proactive strategy that asserts your authority over your circumstances. I must be accountable. I can affect my sickness in a positive way. There are four crucial components to self-help:

- Attitude
- Information
- collaborating with your doctors
- Taking a step

**Attitude**

Studies have shown time and time again that a person's mindset can significantly impact their health. For instance, studies show that those with chronic anger are more prone to experience heart attacks. Our body and thoughts are intertwined. While it's important to eat healthily, exercise, manage stress, and get enough sleep, your attitude may be the most crucial aspect of self-help.

How attitude impacts the physical elements of PD is still unknown. For instance, we are unsure if a positive outlook just reduces symptoms or truly delays the disease's course. We do, however, know that having an optimistic outlook can enhance your quality of life. You might feel better as a result. It may also give you the confidence to adopt the necessary self-care measures to maintain your best possible health for as long as possible.

## Knowledge

Knowledge is yet another crucial self-help tool. You must educate yourself and those close to you on Parkinson's disease (PD) and its causes, symptoms, and available treatments. Keep up with the most recent advancements in science and medicine. Equipping yourselves with knowledge will lessen your anxieties and empower you to make the best-informed medical choices.

## Collaboration with Your Doctors

Self-help does not include acting just on your own behalf. Your doctors must take a significant part in your care since you have a neurological disorder.

An outdated approach to healthcare presupposed that your doctor held absolute authority over you and decided how you would be treated. The self-help paradigm, in contrast, acknowledges that you are an active partner in your health care along with your doctors.

Self-help involves obligations. For example, your doctors must choose the appropriate medication at the appropriate dosage for ailment symptoms. Your responsibility is to take the prescribed dosage on time, monitor your symptoms and side effects, communicate with the doctors about how the drug is functioning, and finally, report any issues you may be experiencing with the recommended course of action.

## Taking Charge

Action implies taking the necessary steps to improve your condition, lessen the effects of your impairment, and maintain your independence for as long as feasible. To improve your diet, take your meds correctly and on time, lessen stress in your life, and get enough sleep, you can apply specific self-help techniques. Each of these tactics will be covered in more detail in the ensuing chapters.

You will give yourself the best opportunity of living better with PD by adopting a positive and cheerful attitude, arming yourself with knowledge, working with your doctors, and taking action.

# Chapter two

# Overview of Parkinson's disease

A degenerative brain illness called Parkinson's disease. Doctors frequently refer to it as a disease of the motor system, the nerve system that regulates body movement.

movement. Parkinson's disease (PD) develops when brain cells, or neurons, deteriorate and result in a lack of the chemical dopamine in the brain. Its chemical (one of the brain's neurotransmitters) has an impact on the area of the brain responsible for motor coordination, attention, learning, and the pleasure and reward system. The signs and symptoms of PD are caused by low dopamine levels.

**Primary Symptoms**

Everybody has a different set of symptoms. For instance, a specific symptom could appear early in one patient but later (or never) in another. The onset of symptoms might be sudden or very gradual. In fact, occasionally the symptoms are mild, and a person may not notice them for weeks or even months. One or both body sides may be affected by the symptoms. A symptom may first appear on one side of the body and then intensify there.

This list of probable symptoms can be concerning. It's crucial to keep in mind that not everyone with PD experiences each symptom listed. Additionally, as was already mentioned, every person experiences PD differently. In addition, the symptoms worsen gradually over time rather than quickly at first.

**Tremor**

The hands, arms, legs, jaw, and head can all tremble.

The typical Parkinson's disease (PD) tremor is characterized by a rhythmic rolling motion between the thumb and forefinger. This tremor is sometimes called "pill rolling" because it resembles the motion of rolling a pill between the fingers and thumb. The hand is where a tremor typically starts, but it can also start in the foot or jaw. In the early stages of the disease, tremor only affects one side of the body in approximately 75% of PD patients. the other 25% of PD patients never experience significant tremor.

**rigidity, or stiffness**

Opposing sets of muscles must alternately relax and contract in order for the body to move smoothly. Muscles in the limbs and trunk may be held stiff and constricted all the time in a person with PD. Aching, stiffness, weakness, and jerky movements could result from it.

**Flow of Movement Is Slow**

Slowness of movement, also known as bradykinesia, is a bothersome and unexpected PD symptom. Simple chores, like dressing, that were once completed quickly may now be time-consuming and difficult.

**Balance and coordination issues**

He may have a stooped posture or be unable to perform various motor skills due to his symptoms if he has Parkinson's disease.

These symptoms usually get worse with time. The individual with PD may eventually have trouble talking, walking, or performing other ordinarily straightforward actions. Additionally, falling is a possibility.

Other potential symptoms include despair and emotional changes. despair in patients with Parkinson's disease is frequent, particularly in the early stages of the illness. drugs for the treatment of PD Sometimes, symptoms make depression worse. Nevertheless, it is safe and effective to combine these medications with some antidepressants.

Fear and insecurity are frequent PD side effects. Some persons with PD may feel they can't handle novel situations and may consequently avoid social events and travel.

**Pain**

According to estimates, almost half of all PD patients deal with some sort of pain. However, patients frequently disregard the discussion of pain as a symptom and believe that it is brought on by other things. Muscle discomfort is a common symptom of PD and can be brought on by bad posture, stiffness, and inactivity; backache is an example of a pain that may stem from these circumstances.

Dystonia, a neurological muscular disease that results in uncontrollable muscle spasms and aberrant movements and postures, may also be a source of pain. It can affect the arms, legs, trunk, neck, face, tongue, jaw, or vocal chords and may be painful. Drugs for Parkinson's disease and exercise both reduce dystonia.

**Loss of memory/slow writing**

Though logic is still apparent, it could be more difficult for someone with PD to recall information or think of solutions as fast as in the past.

## Parkinson's disease

Parkinson's dementia is a more severe mental illness that some people may experience. As you may know, dementia is an illness that affects thinking and memory and is brought on by abnormalities in the brain. Parkinson's disease is known to alter the area of the brain responsible for controlling bodily movements; however, additional brain abnormalities may also have an impact on mental function, leading to dementia. As their condition worsens, it is predicted that 50 to 80 percent of people with Parkinson's disease (PD) would develop dementia; nevertheless, studies have shown that it takes an average of ten years between receiving a PD diagnosis and developing dementia.

## Alzheimer's Psychosis

A serious mood disease called psychosis causes hallucinations or delusions. When something is perceived or heard that is not genuine, it is called a hallucination. Delusions are unfounded beliefs that are unreasonable or irrational. It's estimated that up to 50% of people with PD could experience Parkinson's psychosis. A whopping 80% of people experience visual hallucinations. Auditory (hearing) hallucinations will occur in about 20% of patients. Parkinson's psychosis is a rare occurrence in early-stage Parkinson's disease (PD), typically occurring in advanced stages.

Dementia, depression, sleep issues, decreased vision, and advanced age are risk factors for psychosis. Some PD medicines can exacerbate psychotic symptoms when taken long-term.

Only around 20% of cases of psychosis in PD patients are reported to doctors, making it an underreported and underdiagnosed condition. There could be a number of causes for this. Patients may not want to notify their doctors about their symptoms because they are scared of them or because they are small and barely evident. Some people could be in denial and refuse to admit they are experiencing any symptoms. It is crucial to report such symptoms because once the underlying reason has been identified, there are drugs that could be helpful.

## Swallowing/Chewing Issues

The throat muscles are less effective in the later stages of PD, making it challenging to swallow or chew. Thankfully, drugs can frequently ease these problems.

## Freezing

People with advanced stages of PD frequently experience freezing, a momentary incapacity to move. Movement seems to halt when a "off" switch is pressed. It could be difficult for someone to get out of a chair, or it might feel like their foot is stuck to the floor. Although freezing often only lasts a few seconds or minutes, it can cause falls since it is unpredictable.

## Adaptations in Speech

Rapid speech, slurred or repeated phrases, reluctance when speaking, or speaking too softly or monotonely are all speech alterations that people with PD may encounter. A person with PD may benefit from speech therapy to manage these issues.

## Reduced Smell Sense

In PD patients, the sense of smell is frequently diminished. In fact, research is being done to use the loss of smell as a diagnostic tool for the early detection of PD since doctors think that a compromised sense of smell may be an early predictor of PD. Some people with Parkinson's disease (PD) remember losing some of their sense of smell months or years before other serious PD symptoms appeared.

## Issues urinating or constipation

Some people with PD could experience constipation and have trouble managing their bowels and bladder. As was previously noted, damaged brain neurons impair the proper function of muscles throughout the body, including the digestive system. Additionally, it's conceivable that some of the drugs you take will make you constipated. Constipation can also be relieved by changing one's diet, engaging in regular exercise, and drinking lots of water.

## A Problem Sleeping

People with PD may have trouble falling asleep at night, having nightmares, or remaining asleep. As a result, people could experience daytime sleepiness. Insomnia may be a PD symptom or a side effect of the medications used to treat the disease's symptoms.

## Variations in Expression

A person with PD may have less facial expressions. A person with PD may frown or smile less, and their facial expressions may start to look more "masklike." They may also blink less and seem to gaze. These modifications are the outcome of the intricate adjustments that the body experiences as a result of low dopamine levels.

**Dry/Oily Skin**

People with PD frequently experience greasy or dry skin, excessive sweating, and an extreme sensitivity to heat or cold. Usually, these issues can be resolved with medication and common skin treatments.

**Handwriting changes**

Patients with PD frequently notice changes in their handwriting; it sometimes seems cramped and tiny. Because of the interruption in muscle activity that occurs when not enough dopamine reaches the brain, handwriting changes as a result.

**Stages of PD:** The Course of the Illness

PD affects individuals differently. Some people's sickness advances swiftly. However, the course of the disease is delayed in certain PD patients. Some PD sufferers are severely impaired by their symptoms, while others simply have modest symptoms.

There is a mild "presymptomatic" phase for the majority of PD patients, which may start four to six years before more overt symptoms. A person could experience fatigue or overall malaise. He or she might have some trembling or struggle to get up from a chair. Other early, subtle signs could be:

minor weakened state of an extremity

when walking, one leg feels stiff

minimal trembling

mood shifts

alterations in posture

reduced ability to smell

memory issues

dizziness

alterations to handwriting

alterations in speech

joint and muscle discomfort

Frequently, the condition starts off as a brief tremor that comes and goes. However, the tremor could increase in frequency and eventually cover the entire arm. Arm rigidity or stiffness may then occur. Simple chores like buttoning garments could get challenging. The affected leg becomes stiffer and more difficult to move over time.

Most of the time, these changes are so minor or gradual that nobody really notices them. Frequently, a person's loved ones' relatives or friends are the first to notice a change in them.

The symptoms could become worse as the years go by. Both sides of the body may experience the tremor and rigidity. Movement might slow down. One's expression loses its lively quality.

It is simple to understand how stiff limbs, sluggish mobility, and a shuffling stride may be mistaken for typical, aging-related changes, particularly in older persons. Sometimes the exhaustion and lack of facial expression lead to a mistaken diagnosis of depression. Many persons with PD and their loved ones dismiss the early symptoms as "old age." It may take some time before the symptoms start to interfere to the point where one feels the need to seek medical attention because they frequently develop slowly over many years.

PD symptoms are divided into stages by doctors. The following is a description of each stage, such as when your doctor says, "You have stage 1 Parkinson's disease."

## Parkinson's disease stages

### Stage 1

Only one side of the body is affected by the signs and symptoms. (Symptoms are what a patient experiences; signs are what a doctor observes.)

**Mild symptoms exist.**

Although uncomfortable, symptoms are not incapacitating.

Typically, a tremor only affects one limb.

Changes in posture, movement, and facial expression are observed by friends and other close people.

### Stage 2

Both sides of the body experience the symptoms.

Symptoms only slightly impair people.

Gait and posture are impacted.

## Stage 3

Movements of the body are noticeably slowed.

Moderate to severe difficulties with daily functioning are brought on by symptoms.

## Stage 4

The signs are quite bad.

A person can still walk, but only to a certain degree.

Rigidity and are experienced by certain patients.

sluggishness of motion.

Patient is unable to live alone any longer.

Neurologists classify a fifth stage as one in which a patient's debilitation necessitates confinement to a bed or wheelchair. For many patients, early self-care and medication therapy may postpone this stage of the disease until very late in the course of it or even completely prevent it.

## Who Develops PD?

I got PD, why did that happen?"Nobody truly knows. However, you are not alone. About 2% of people over sixty-one have Parkinson's disease. In children and young adults, it is unusual but not unheard of. All ethnic groups and both men and women are equally susceptible to PD.

Every year, the United States alone diagnoses over 60,000 new cases. Research indicates that there may be twice as many undiagnosed cases of Parkinson's disease as the one million or more cases that have received a diagnosis in the United States. By 2030, the prevalence of PD is anticipated to double.

PD is more prevalent than multiple sclerosis, muscular dystrophy, and amyotrophic lateral sclerosis in terms of patient population (Loucoupled with Gehrig's illness).

## What Leads to PD?

It is unknown what specifically causes Parkinson's disease. Researchers have found hints regarding the causes, though. It is obvious that a deficiency in the brain chemical dopamine has a significant role.

There are various hypotheses regarding potential reasons.

## Nerve cell injury

Parkinson's disease is brought on by the progressive degeneration of dopamine-producing brain nerve cells. As was already established, normal nerve function is affected when this chemical's production is impeded, which in turn affects how well movements are coordinated. Why these nerve cells degenerate is a mystery to medical researchers.

## Radical Freethinkers

There may be additional causes of PD. Free radicals, commonly known as oxidants, may harm or destroy nerve cells and cause PD, according to some researchers. Free radicals are incredibly unstable chemicals that the body naturally produces during normal metabolism.

Only when there are more free radicals than the body can handle can they destroy cells.

Vitamins A, C, and E are antioxidants that combat free radicals. Damage from free radicals occurs when your body creates an excessive quantity of them owing to stress, drug or alcohol addiction, smoking, sun damage, or a variety of other circumstances. It also happens when your intake of antioxidants (from food or supplements) is too low. Free radicals can cause a variety of diseases, including Parkinson's, heart disease, and cancer.

**Describe Parkinsonism.**

A collection of movement disorders with symptoms resembling those of Parkinson's disease are referred to as Parkinsonism, sometimes known as Parkinson's syndrome or parkinsonian syndrome. It describes illnesses that exhibit symptoms similar to those of Parkinson's disease but are brought on by other underlying causes.

Parkinsonism can be brought on by a variety of factors, such as certain drugs, brain damage, infections, poisons, or other neurological degenerative disorders. These diseases may produce tremors, bradykinesia (slowness of movement), rigidity (stiffness), and postural instability (difficulty maintaining balance), which are motor symptoms resembling Parkinson's disease.

It is essential to distinguish between Parkinson's disease and parkinsonism since the prognosis and course of treatment may vary depending on the underlying cause. A specific type of neurological ailment called Parkinson's disease is characterized by a progressive loss of dopamine-producing brain cells. Parkinsonism, on the other hand, covers a wider variety of ailments with symptoms similar to Parkinson's brought on by many causes.

**toxins in the environment**

Many experts think that internal or external poisons might kill brain nerve cells that carry dopamine. A designer drug called MPTP that was a kind of synthetic morphine was available on the streets in the 1980s. It turns out that the drug was known to cause some drug users to develop PD symptoms quite quickly.

Similar to this, some scientists contend that dopamine-producing brain cells may be harmed by drug interactions as well as by exposure to toxins including pesticides, carbon monoxide, heavy metals, or toxins in the food supply. Dopamine is a brain neurotransmitter that is necessary to prevent the symptoms of Parkinson's disease (PD).

## Increased Aging

According to another view, PD symptoms develop when the normal, age-related loss of dopamine-producing neurons accelerates. It is unknown what is causing this accelerated aging.

## Genetic Variables

According to a recently proposed notion, PD susceptibility may be inherited. Multiple occurrences of PD in one family are uncommon, although they do occur. The likelihood of your offspring developing PD is relatively low if there is no clear family history.

## Use of Specific Drugs

As previously indicated, several medicines may result in a PD-like condition that is typically reversible. For instance, risperidone-containing blood pressure medications and tranquilizers like haloperidol, thioridazine, and chlorpromazine may interfere with dopamine in the brain and result in PD symptoms. A kind of Parkinsonism may also result from the extended use of antipsychotic (neuroleptic) medications, such as those prescribed to treat schizophrenia, however this side effect is reversible if the medication is stopped.

## How is PD identified?

Parkinson's disease may be challenging to diagnose in its early stages. Early symptoms could be hazy and unrelated at first. They could appear and disappear suddenly. As was already mentioned, symptoms of PD might be mistaken for aging-related changes or for signs of other nerve conditions.

**clinical assessment**

The most frequent methods used by doctors to make the diagnosis of Parkinson's disease are a clinical examination and the gathering of a patient's medical history. A clinical examination may reveal physical signs such as stiffness, tremor at rest, slowness of movement, and shuffling. Memory loss, loss of smell, constipation, and autonomic dysfunction—issues with things like blood pressure, heart rate, perspiration, and food digestion—are examples of other neurological (nonmotor) symptoms.

Even for a neurologist who is knowledgeable with the condition, it can occasionally be challenging to accurately diagnose PD given the patient's history and physical examination.

A doctor might advise trying out anti-Parkinson's medications. If symptoms improve while taking the medication, it is a clinical sign that PD may be the origin of the issue; however, if symptoms do not improve, the issue may be brought on by another sort of neurological disorder.

## Diagnostic imaging's function

A doctor may request a particular diagnostic scan known as a SPECT scan (single-photon emission computed tomography) to help support a PD diagnosis. Due to the use of a radiopharmaceutical, also known as a radioactive tracer, and a specialized camera, it is known as a nuclear imaging test. The camera's images demonstrate how interior organs and tissues function. A doctor might request a nuclear imaging SPECT exam with DaTscan, the radioactive tracer, in order to better understand what might be causing Parkinson's-related symptoms. DaT, which stands for "dopamine transporter," is the first radioactive tracer that the FDA has approved for use in enabling doctors to view computer graphics that display a patient's brain's dopamine transporter status.

Remember that a lack of the brain chemical dopamine plays a part in the movement abnormalities brought on by Parkinson's disease to better appreciate why this scan is beneficial. The SPECT scan with DaTscan evaluates the quantity and distribution of the tracer in the brain and can reveal information on the relative health of the dopamine system in the region of the brain connected to movement by detecting the dopamine transporters on the dopamine neurons.

it in turn provides information to the doctor on the condition of the dopamine-producing brain cells.

having a SPECT scan done. If you have one of these scans booked, plan on spending the majority of the day at the radiology department of the hospital or clinic where it will be done; the entire process will take about six hours. You will be urged to drink plenty of water before the scan in order to stay hydrated. Put on relaxed clothing.

The intravenous (IV) injection of DaTscan radiopharmaceutical will be given to you in the arm. After the injection, the tracer must pass through your body before it can go to the parts of your brain that will be scanned. Before the test can start, you'll have to wait three to six hours. During this period, you're free to roam around and can even leave the imaging facility and come back later.

You will be asked to lie on a table so that you can be scanned after the tracer has had a chance to circulate. The radioactive tracer in your brain is detected by a sizable, spherical gadget called a SPECT machine. The device has a unique camera that will be placed over your head. Since it's crucial that you keep your head still throughout the treatment, a technician will probably put on a chin strap to do just that.

En, a camera gently circles your head for about 30 minutes while detecting the radioactive tracer and sending the data to a computer to produce photos. We will only scan your head in part, from the top of your ears.

When you urinate after your scan, the radioactive tracer will be removed from your body. Your doctor could advise you to consume more fluids to aid in the removal of the tracer from your body. Within a few days, your body ought to have entirely eliminated the tracer.

Your scan's findings. When your results will be available, ask your doctor. Your doctor will examine the images generated by your scan in order to interpret the findings. The colors or gradations of grey in the photographs will indicate to your doctor which regions of your brain absorbed more radioactive tracer and which regions absorbed less.

The tracer will display crescent-shaped patterns on both sides of the brain if the scan results are normal; such a pattern would not suggest the presence of a degenerative disease like Parkinson's. However, an aberrant scan, brought on by a lack of dopamine, will show up as circular or oval shapes on one or both sides of the brain in the scan results. It is a sign of Parkinson's disease or perhaps another neurological condition that is connected to it. Examples of both normal and abnormal brain scan results.

It is crucial that a qualified doctor with nuclear medicine training administers and interprets your scan. The first step for a professional is to establish whether the scan is normal or abnormal. He or she will then decide if the scan results exhibit Parkinson's disease-like symptoms.

## Recognizing Your Diagnoses

If you're like the majority of people, you'll find it difficult to comprehend that you have a long-term, degenerative condition like Parkinson's. You might want to confirm the diagnosis with more information.

If necessary, seek a second and even third opinion. If one doctor diagnoses you with PD, you can start to doubt that doctor's judgment. However, it is more difficult to dispute a PD diagnosis if two or three medical professionals agree with it.

Regarding your symptoms, be honest. How long have you been off-balance? List all of the symptoms you have observed. then go through the list. Do you have any of the "classic" PD symptoms like tremor, sluggishness, or stiffness?

Obtain feedback from loved ones by asking them. What signs have they seen? Have they seen any more changes?

Find out what causes Parkinson's disease and what you can do to prevent it. As you'll discover as you read this book, there are medicines that are quite effective in treating Parkinson's disease. You'll also discover that there are ways to put in place assistance systems.

**One last word on symptoms**

It makes sense that receiving a PD diagnosis can be worrisome. But keep in mind that not everyone experiences every symptom. It's crucial to keep in mind that PD symptoms never suddenly get worse; rather, they always worsen over time. If your symptoms appear suddenly, they may be caused by another medical condition, such as an infection like a urinary tract infection (UTI), which is more prevalent in older women. Additionally, certain symptoms that arise unexpectedly can be caused by a prescription change. Naturally, you'll want to discuss any such symptoms with your doctor.

Finally, you will discover the numerous medications that can help reduce PD symptoms in the chapters that follow. Additionally, you'll discover fresh approaches to managing a chronic illness.

# Chapter three

# Parkinson's Disease: Its Emotional Impact

Chronic, long-term illnesses like Parkinson's disease (PD) can strain marriages, alienate friends and friendships, and deplete hard-earned financial resources.

resources. Finding out you have PD can be disastrous. You might experience emotions like rage, regret, remorse, and fear. You can reject that you have the condition, withdraw, or experience depression. The fact that these emotions and responses are natural is among the most crucial things to understand. Most persons with PD go through some or all of them at some point in their lives.

When receiving such news, there is no right or wrong, good or poor response. You cannot be told how to respond by anyone. Your response to the illness and how you handle it will shape and color your life and, to a lesser extent, the lives of those you care about.

## Getting Past Denial

People often become unknowingly affected by PD as it develops slowly and invisibly. You may have ignored your symptoms, denying any, but prior to diagnosis, you probably knew you were "not quite yourself."

For as long as you could, there was a major problem.

This response is both typical and common. Self-defense is a sort of denial. We are never willing to acknowledge a significant problem. You probably found yourself vacillating between denial of any issue and concern and worry about what the issue might be before your diagnosis. The mental stress and worry undoubtedly got worse as your illnesses got worse and you had greater physical limits.

If you're like most individuals, it makes sense that receiving a PD diagnosis might distress you. You recently learned that you have a chronic, incapacitating illness. However, it is somewhat relieving to finally have a term for your nebulous symptoms.

But all of a sudden, your future becomes hazy. You start to wonder: What will I be able to do? Is it still possible to work? Am I still capable of being a parent or a partner? What kinds of medical expenses will I be responsible for?

Refusing to accept a PD diagnosis is not unusual. Unfortunately, denial requires a lot of effort and creates stress. If you try to conceal your symptoms, you could feel isolated and embarrassed. The sooner you accept your condition, the sooner you can start dealing with it and living your life. As long as you deny the disease, you remain its unsuspecting victim.

**Getting Rid of Unfounded Fears**

Before there were effective treatments like levodopa (l-dopa), when PD was more disabling and less treatable than it is now, you might have encountered friends, relatives, or acquaintances who were diagnosed with the condition. Fortunately, there are currently effective drug treatments for many PD symptoms.

Here are a few strategies to dispel unwarranted worries and stop your imagination from upsetting you excessively:

**Find a medical professional with whom you can communicate:** Find someone who will discuss your worries and fears with you.

**Do all you can to learn about the illness:** Study a book. Investigate information about websites that publish trustworthy information.

**With your doctor, family, and encouraging friends, discuss your anxietie:** To "air" your anxieties is beneficial. Your anxieties become less intimidating when you face them head-on.

**Be a part of a PD support group:** Members of such organizations can share information about the most recent treatments, suggest doctors, and offer practical coping strategies in addition to friendship and moral support.

**Consult a mental health professional:** Consult a mental-health expert if you've tried all of these tips but are still feeling stressed out.

## Getting Yourself Back in Control

When given a PD diagnosis, the question "Why me? Your life appears to be spiraling out of control all of a sudden. Even if you make every effort to control your life, there will inevitably be times when you feel powerless. You have no control over a slippery, icy stretch of the road, a mechanical issue with the airplane you're flying, or the fact that your brain's dopamine levels are low.

Your enthusiasm and energy are sapped when you view yourself as a victim, and you begin to feel too reliant on other people.

The good news is that you can reclaim control over your life.

Although you have no control over your PD, you do have a lot of control over how it affects your life.

Your concerns can be allayed and your sense of independence can be restored by learning about PD. Think about the following to get your bearings:

**Don't just accept your doctor's advice passively;** take an active role in your healthcare. Pose inquiries. Ask questions till you comprehend if you don't. Make recommendations.

**Keep your independence as much as you can:** Some people who have chronic illnesses respond by becoming more and more reliant on others. These people with PD may eventually lose their ability to function, not because of the illness itself but because of their emotional responses to it. Do as much of your own work as you can instead, and only seek assistance when absolutely necessary.

**Plan ahead:** Work together with your doctor to create an efficient treatment strategy. Make a list of all the self-care activities you can engage in, such as regular exercise, healthy food, stress management, and medication administration.

## Taking back one's sense of self

I, who am I? You might be curious: You are greater than your illness, rest assured. You may not be as capable of carrying out daily tasks as you were before being diagnosed with PD, but you are still an important person. The following advice will help you strengthen your personal defenses and restore your sense of self.

Learn to accept assistance when you truly need it: It can be challenging to rely on others, but your illness will prevent you from performing some tasks. You'll need assistance. Without sacrificing your dignity, learn to accept this greater degree of need.

Learn to deal with people's unfavorable reactions: You may occasionally have to put up with others being unkind or insensitive, especially strangers. If people glare, display animosity, pity, or rejection, put it down to their lack of understanding of this complicated illness.

Discuss coping strategies with others: People who have chronic illnesses have been in your shoes and understand how you feel. You might feel less isolated and different by communicating with them and exchanging feelings, thoughts, and ideas.

Recall your prior victories: This advice does not imply wallowing in regret or lamenting the past. Just keep in mind all of your prior accomplishments, accolades, and successes since they can lift your spirits when you're depressed.

Pay attention to the tiny wins since they add up over time rather than the big ones. Establish objectives and record your accomplishments. To keep your spirits high, think about keeping a written or audio journal of your victories and reviewing it frequently.

Avoid lash outs: Your illness may make you angry at times. Especially your loved ones and caretakers, refrain from venting your anger on them.

Steer clear of destructive habits: Some people abuse alcohol and drugs to dull the pain of difficult difficulties like chronic sickness. These "fixes" are only short-term, and they will ultimately make your disease harder to manage.

## Getting Over Depression

About half of patients with PD experience depression, which is typical with the disorder. The "blues" that the majority of us occasionally experience are not the same as depression, which is a more serious condition. The following are some signs of depression:

**feeling down**

- reduced enjoyment or interest in activities
- without dieting or weight gain, weight loss
- a lack of sleep or excessive sleep

- either becoming agitated or sluggish

- exhaustion or a lack of energy

- Sense of insignificance

- reduced capacity for thought or concentration

- persistent suicidal or death thoughts

You may be depressed if you encounter several of these signs and symptoms for two weeks or more. Although mild sadness is the norm for people with Parkinson's disease, some have moderate or even severe depression.

Some PD patients' brains may undergo metabolic alterations that contribute to depression: Serotonin, a brain chemical thought to be crucial in the control of mood, has been found to be lower in persons with depression, according to studies. Endogenous depression is the term used by doctors to describe this biochemical imbalance in the brain, which can be fatal if left untreated.

Depression may also be brought on by PD medications: Typically, in the first two weeks following the initiation of pharmacological treatment, anxiety, restlessness, or worry precedes depression brought on by PD medicines. After this time, you can have mood fluctuations, insomnia, or both for a few weeks. After five or six weeks, symptoms typically reach their height as the body becomes used to the medicine and the depression starts to subside. If you suspect your depression is due to the medications you are taking, consult with your doctor. It could be possible to alter your prescription or dosage.

The symptoms of depression that are also present in PD, such as weariness, sluggishness, sleeplessness, and difficulty concentrating, can lead to confusion or incorrect diagnoses when it comes to PD-related depression. Depression may first conceal PD symptoms. Later, depression may be concealed by PD symptoms.

It's crucial to get treatment for depression symptoms if you have them. Antidepressant drugs can be recommended by your doctor, and they may also help with other PD symptoms. Here are some additional ideas to improve your mood:

*Get moving:* The body naturally elevates mood by releasing endorphins when you move. If you are unable to complete an assignment

Do something else if you're feeling "off" or exhausted. The secret is to keep yourself as active as you can, both physically and mentally.

Set modest, defined goals that are realistic and attainable to prevent depressive feelings from overwhelming you. Set a deadline for each objective. Set objectives in all areas of your life, including physical activity, job, social interactions, spiritual development, and leisure pursuits like crafts that will hone your motor skills. Your list of objectives might resemble this:

- Spend at least fifteen minutes each day working out.
- Participate once a week in a PD support group.
- this month, consider taking an online course.

Avoid being critical of oneself: When you're depressed, it's simple to criticize yourself. Refocus your attention on your successes whenever you hear that inner voice saying something negative, such as "I'm too slow" or "I used to be able to do this, but now I can't." Substitute positive statements like "I do my job well," "I'm a great parent," or "I have a good relationship with my family" for negative ones.

Keep in touch with people: People with Parkinson's disease (PD) in the early stages frequently experience embarrassment over their symptoms, particularly tremors. You could feel uneasy in social settings if moving around is difficult or awkward for you. You could isolate yourself from others and forgo your typical social and leisure activities out of fear of looking foolish.

Staying connected is crucial for your mental and emotional wellness because isolation only makes depression worse. By engaging in religious activities, hosting events, taking lessons, visiting friends, volunteering, and attending support group meetings, you can increase your chances of meeting new people.

Share your thoughts, feelings, anxieties, worries, goals, and dreams with friends and loved ones by talking about them. Do not be ashamed to express your feelings of isolation, shame, rage, and frustration. You might be shocked to find how opening up about your inner sentiments can strengthen your bonds with others.

Try counseling: If these methods are ineffective in relieving your symptoms, think about seeking more help by speaking with a mental-health counselor.

**decreasing stress**

Stress frequently exacerbates PD symptoms, particularly tremors. PD has not been linked to stress as a cause, however stress can exacerbate or even start symptoms. It's critical to manage stress well.

Determine the origins of your stress. Everybody experiences stress in different ways. Even enjoyable circumstances can be stressful. Social occasions may increase symptoms and induce worry for many people with PD, particularly those who have just been diagnosed, adding to their stress. Instead of avoiding social events and isolating yourself, consider what adjustments you might make to lessen the stress. Make a list of the issues that stress you out.

Create and stick to a stress-reduction plan. For instance, perhaps you had trouble slicing the meat on your last lunch with friends, and numerous portions of your meal ended up on the floor. You vowed to turn down similar invites in the future since you felt degraded and embarrassed.

Ask yourself instead, "How could I approach this differently? How might I manage my condition while still having a good time at lunch with my friends?Ordering a meal that doesn't require the ability to cut meat, asking a friend to help you chop your meat, or requesting the waitress to cut your share into bite-sized pieces before bringing it to the table are all potential alternatives.

Adapt your expectations: Trying to perform intellectually and physically in the same manner as you once did could cause excessive anxiety.

Reprioritize: A life-changing illness makes you rethink your priorities. What matters most to you?

Spending more time with your granddaughter or making one more sale? Is it increasing your income or giving your time to a subject you're passionate about? What's most significant is up to you to determine.

This kind of introspection might lead to you switching careers or lowering your housekeeping standards. Your revised priorities might help you discover more about who you really are and what makes you happy.

Set objectives. Make sure that your objectives are both reachable and tough so that they will cause you to "stretch" a little. Spend some time establishing goals for your social, spiritual, physical, financial, and other areas of life. Set both short-term and long-term goals each week.

Many of us are in a time pressure, so schedule your time to prevent tense deadlines. We frequently race to make appointments, barely arriving on time. Give everything more time. When scheduling appointments, try to be as accurate as you can so that you don't arrive late.

Sleep well: Plan your day as much as you can to allow for extra rest following a very active day. If your way of life let you, restfully nap every afternoon. Short afternoon naps (less than forty minutes) have been demonstrated in research to (Five minutes) can help you feel more at ease, rested, and awake.

Caffeine should be consumed in moderation because it might cause jitteriness. Caffeine can be found in chocolate, black tea, cola, and other drinks. Drink decaf variations or restrict your daily caffeine intake to one cup. Before turning in for the evening, stay away from caffeine-containing beverages.

Create processes to make it easier for you to find stuff and get organized. Every day, set goods in the same location. You won't have to worry about not being able to find your wallet, pocketbook, or keys, for example, especially if you have to find them quickly.

As previously noted, no one likes feeling dependent. But for some tasks, you will need the help of family and friends. Asking for help from others enables you to be open and vulnerable while also enabling them to provide you with the gift of assistance. Although it could be challenging at first, interdependence can eventually bring individuals together.

Practice deep breathing by remaining still and closing your eyes. Inhale deeply while counting to four, filling both your lungs and your abdomen. then gradually let it go. For five or six breaths, repeat.

Relax gradually by finding a peaceful spot to sit or lie down where you won't be disturbed. Groups of muscles should be tensed and then released, beginning with the head. As you move down your body, gradually tense and release your muscles. When you have fully tightened and then released, sit or lie still for several minutes.

Think about joining a meditation class. Alternately, try this easy meditation technique: Take a seat quietly, close your eyes, and breathe normally. Think of the word "one" (or "peace" or "calm") each time you inhale. When thoughts arise, simply let them go and slowly bring your attention back to your word and breathing. Keep going for 10 to 15 minutes.

Many thoughts, or so-called "monkey mind," when your mind seems to leap from one thought to the next, may first upset you. Not to worry. With time and repetition, you'll discover that you can relax and savor the tranquil solitude more easily. Every time you feel worn out or overburdened, whether in the morning or the early evening, take a meditation break.

Yoga might help you to stay more flexible and relax your thoughts. Deep breathing, moderate stretching, and strengthening are all components of many postures.

Investigate biofeedback: In this exercise, you will discover how to use visual or aural stimuli to control your own bodily functions. The skills must first be learned from a doctor or a biofeedback technician. But once you know them, you'll surely feel more in charge of your body and stress levels.

Relax with guided imagery: Hundreds of recordings are available for purchase or loan from the library that combine soothing sounds or music with instructions for a fictitious "trip." For example, guided imagery might involve imagining yourself lying in a green meadow where you can smell the flowers, hear the gentle twitter of birds, and feel the sun warming your body. You will be able to envision on your own and take a brief "mental vacation" whenever necessary once you get used to using these recordings.

## Informing Others of Your Illness

Informing people about your PD could make you anxious and stressed out. How soon should you inform others? Should you inform anyone? Do you need to notify your boss? Do you have any grandchildren or children? Which details should you share?

These questions have no right or wrong answers. To avoid questioning, some people choose to tell everyone they know. Others decide to keep their symptoms a secret from everyone until they become obvious. These are questions that you must answer for yourself.

*One thing is certain:* Trying to conceal your illness will only make you more nervous, especially if symptoms get worse. Your symptoms can then get worse due to anxiety. Medical professionals have discovered that those who are able to acknowledge their illness and share it with others do the best. Remember that PD affects not just you but also everyone in your immediate family. Everyone in your social network must support you, be understanding, and help you to effectively manage and treat PD. It is more difficult to start the process of accepting your sickness if you keep it hidden. Here are some broad pointers for disclosing your disease to loved ones, friends, acquaintances, coworkers, employers, and others:

*Once you've decided who to tell, be honest and upfront;* there's no point in trying to sugarcoat the situation. Before alerting coworkers at work, it's a good idea to discuss it with your boss.

Don't wait too long to let people know how they can help, especially when your needs change. If your symptoms are obvious, friends and coworkers will naturally wonder what's wrong and will likely come up with an incorrect "diagnosis."

*Help others understand PD:* Some individuals, particularly those close to you, may need to learn more about PD. Learning about the condition might reassure them that many people with PD have active, fulfilling lives. You can find a ton of material from many sources online or in print, and you can also get information in the library and online.

Having conversations with your partner
Your partner is virtually equally impacted by a chronic illness as you are. If he or she isn't there when you get the PD diagnosis, it's crucial that you tell them as soon as you can.

Any chronic condition can put extreme strain on a marriage or other long-term partnership. A Parkinson's disease diagnosis could be troublesome if the relationship is already in jeopardy. The realities of a long-term sickness might not be something your partner can or wants to deal with. Negative emotions could include denial, anger or resentment over potential changes to important relationship tenets, such as established roles, and fear and overprotectiveness, when they always feel the need to "take care" of you. These reactions, while entirely acceptable and very typical, are not helpful.

If you're fortunate enough to be in a committed relationship, the PD diagnosis may put your relationship to the test but won't have any negative effects. Instead, it might eventually bring the two of you closer together.

One of the most challenging aspects of PD is having to deal with your partner's reactions. However, it's crucial to avoid letting your partner's responses worsen your symptoms. Here are some methods for assisting your companion:

Don't sugar-coat your prognosis to appease your partner; instead, be open and honest about your situation. Similarly, avoid making things look more severe than it is. You both deserve to be fully and honestly informed because you are in this together.

Accept the responses they give. It's important to keep in mind that there is no one "right" way for a spouse to react to such life-altering news.

Reassure your partner by telling them that most people with Parkinson's disease live long, fulfilling lives with therapy and that the majority, if not all, of their symptoms can be managed.

Keep your independence as much as you can. Be practical: Ask for assistance when you need it, but avoid becoming unduly reliant.
It's challenging to provide care; your partner already has plenty to worry about.

Encourage your partner to actively engage with the healthcare team; this will make you both feel like you're in this together.

Together, the partners should acquire resources about PD and learn as much as they can about the illness.

Encourage your partner to go to caregiver support groups: Many towns provide partner-caregivers support groups where they may express their emotions, obtain helpful coping strategies, and feel less alone.

Support your partner's extracurricular activities and relationships: It's crucial for your partner to pursue and maintain personal interests, including hobbies, classes, sports, clubs, and activities related to their religion or community. If your partner isn't completely consumed with you and your condition, he or she will experience less stress and provide greater care.

Discuss your finances openly: The lack of money is one of the major worries a partner has when their partner is ill. Sit down and evaluate your financial condition honestly. Examine your medical coverage. Create a sensible budget. Could you reduce some costs to save money? Look into federal financial aid programs if necessary.

Determine your network of support: Who else in your sphere of relatives and friends can you rely on for assistance? Full-time partner carers require assistance and breaks. Who else can take you to the doctor if your partner can't?

Talk, talk, talk: Effective PD coping and harmonious relationship maintenance depend on close communication. An effective communication strategy can be the difference between a partnership that survives adversity and one that deteriorates.

**conversing with kids**

Children must eventually be told as well. Here are some pointers for discussing your illness with kids.

Use language that is appropriate for the child's age. Too much or too little information delivered in a way that appears ominous or menacing may inspire fantasies and anxieties in kids. Avoid making predictions about the future; instead, describe your grandmother's condition to young children by saying, "Grandmother has a sickness that causes her hands to tremble," or yourself, "I have a nerve problem that causes my hands to tremble." You might need to provide further details when the issue worsens.

Kids are great at asking direct questions, especially if you let them know it's okay to talk about your health. So, encourage kids to do so. "Grandpa, why don't you stand up straight?""Mommy, why don't you smile?""Aunt Mary, why is your voice so soft?"

Let kids express their worries; keeping them bottled up can lead to irrational fears. Make a friendly space where children can express their fears, anxieties, and worries about the situation.

Reassure kids by saying that your illness is not fatal and that it is not contagious. Children frequently worry that they could "catch" someone else's health issues. Explain to older kids that the majority of research indicates that PD is not an inherited condition. Additionally, reassure them that neither they nor anybody else did anything to cause you to develop the illness.

Maintain a casual, conversational tone; if you weep or exhibit signs of tension, youngsters may worry needlessly. They will be able to maintain perspective if you approach PD with calm and objectivity. Children will accept you more for who you are if you are more accepting of your situation.

Use humor: Funny things can frequently make uncomfortable situations bearable. Children will be able to tell if you are using comedy to cover up reality or your true emotions. But the situation is easier to handle when you can laugh at yourself and your circumstance.

**Disclosing to Your Employer**

Informing an employer is not a problem because some people with PD receive their diagnosis after they have retired. When they are diagnosed, other people are still working, though. Do I need to tell my employer?" is a common query from those who have just received a PD diagnosis. A more practical query may be, "When should I inform my employer?"

Unfortunately, there isn't a straightforward answer. Every situation is different. When you must inform your manager will depend on the type of employment you have. An airplane pilot or a brain surgeon, for example, will probably need to inform their company more quickly than an insurance salesperson. When you inform your employer will also depend on how quickly your illness is progressing, how effectively your symptoms can be managed with medicine, and how well you get along with your boss and the business.

Nobody can foresee what will happen after telling an employer. Your boss may be understanding regarding your doctor's appointments and make modifications to your workplace to facilitate your task. Different bosses show less compassion. You can be forced into an early retirement or given new responsibilities at work.

Keep in mind that PD is a handicap. Despite the fact that it may be challenging and expensive to succeed in such a legal battle, you are protected by federal law from being classified as red just because you have PD. Before speaking with your employer, take into account the following:

Talk freely with your doctors about your employment position and any restrictions at the office.

Consult your doctors about any modifications that can allow you to keep up your productivity at work.

List the benefits and drawbacks of telling your employer. Ask yourself, "Can I still do this job and do it well? " after taking a realistic look at your circumstances."

Offer your employer some recommendations regarding accommodations. Perhaps you can work from home, like many people who do so these days.

**Finding Focus and Adjusting to Changing Roles**
PD will inevitably alter your roles at both work and home. It's likely to alter your perception of oneself as well. It's crucial to remember that you are not your illness. You happen to have Parkinson's disease. Simply said, your illness is a component of who you are.

You might not be able to do your typical tasks at home, which could have an impact on how you feel about yourself. Your partner and kids might start doing things that you used to do alone or together, like driving, paying bills, making choices, and organizing social events.

Driving a car is the ultimate symbol of independence for some people. However, it's critical for people with PD to be realistic about their capacity to continue driving due to changes in motor and focus skills. Some PD patients voluntarily renounce their driver's license. Some people are insistent that they should keep this emblem of their freedom. At some point, it will be critical to decide whether it is still safe for you to drive by having a professional driving teacher evaluate your driving abilities.

We have mainly discussed dealing with losses in this chapter. But what would you substitute for those losses? You must set new priorities and give your life new direction and significance.

Many of us feel that our jobs define who we are. We don't say, "I'm a loving, loyal person," but rather, "I'm a doctor" (or "I'm a lawyer," or "I'm a secretary," or "I'm a teacher," etc.). When that work role changes or vanishes, we can be at a loss.

Not everyone who has PD must leave their vocation. Many people can still function well. Keep working as long as you can if you can still do your job competently. Look for ways to shift jobs or make modifications that would allow you to continue working if changes in your physical and mental capacities make it difficult for you to continue in your current position. You might be able to work remotely using technology like computers, fax machines, cell phones, and other tools, as discussed before.

If your current job gets too challenging, think about switching careers. Look at your background and abilities. How can you use them in a different capacity? Maybe you might find a less stressful part-time job or work as a consultant.

The goal is to continue working and making a difference for as long as you are able.

Not everyone is able to or want to keep working. Many persons who develop PD are close to or already retired and would prefer to pursue other interests. That is acceptable as long as you feel focused, purposeful, fulfilled, and accomplished when engaging in those activities. Perhaps by getting active in church, community, or volunteer work, you can change your attention from your own difficulties to those of others. Or, for a fulfilling experience, think about enrolling in or instructing a class for adults or kids in a subject of interest.

# Chapter four

# Your Physician as a Partner

Maintaining a positive relationship with your doctors is essential when you have a chronic illness like Parkinson's disease. After all, you and your medical professionals will likely manage your condition together for years to come.

Many of us were brought up thinking that doctors were somehow magical, that their advice was always correct, and that the patient's job was to simply follow the doctor's instructions without question. The times have evolved. You must build and keep a strong collaboration with your doctors in order to meet the demands of a complex and difficult disease like Parkinson's disease. To the cooperation, each of you will contribute knowledge and skills.

The medical and clinical expertise will be provided by your doctors and other members of your health care team. You will provide knowledge of how you feel physically and emotionally, as well as how those feelings evolve over time. You have the right to query any drug or operation your doctor suggests as a partner in your healthcare. You are also entitled to a second opinion. Decisions regarding your care must be made collaboratively by you and your doctors. You will be given the finest care possible for your condition if you have a good collaboration.

**Team for Your Health Care**

A primary care physician and a neurologist are often the least two doctors that PD patients see. Your "regular" doctor, sometimes known as your family doctor, is a primary-care physician.

A primary-care doctor is typically an internist, a family doctor, or a general practitioner.

You'll most likely be sent to a neurologist by your primary care physician. Your primary-care doctor might monitor and treat your disease as well as any additional health issues when they arise, depending on your condition and your medical insurance plan.

Your insurance policy might only let you visit a neurologist or other expert on occasion.

A physician who specializes in the diagnosis and treatment of nervous system conditions is known as a neurologist. You should get a neurologist evaluation because PD is a nervous-system disorder. Ideally, your neurologist will diagnose or confirm PD, offer a course of treatment, and keep an eye on it.

Like many other medical professionals, neurologists may have diverse interests and backgrounds. The phrase "movement disorders" refers to a subspecialty of neurology that includes illnesses with movement-related symptoms. Some neurologists continue their education in this field. Some even continue working as researchers and clinicians in PD research facilities housed in universities. If one of these research centers exists in your area, you can locate trained neurologists there. Look for a neurologist in your area who is interested in, trained in, and experienced in treating PD patients.

You might require additional specialty care depending on your symptoms. For instance, some PD sufferers report mental abnormalities, including challenging thoughts, feelings, and behaviors as well as memory loss. Diagnose and treat mental problems only by a psychiatrist, a medical professional with specialized training in mental health. To treat mental health concerns brought on by PD, he or she may turn to psychotherapy, marital counseling, and family therapy, in addition to medicine. A psychiatrist may initially consult with you before referring you to another mental-health professional, like a clinical psychologist or a social worker, for longer-term care.

Frequently, families that have loved ones with PD have a wide range of requirements, including material, psychological, and social needs. A social worker who has received training in family and marriage therapy may also be able to assist you in finding other community services. Psychiatrists frequently charge more than such service providers.

Your health insurance plan may also affect who you visit.)

Your doctor might suggest that you see an occupational therapist if you are struggling with self-care, work, or leisure activities. This expert can assist you in making equipment selections that will safely help you manage many of your symptoms and make life easier.

Your mobility, posture, and balance issues can be handled by a physical therapist. He or she is qualified to evaluate such physical issues and suggest the right activities. Additionally, a physical therapist can assist you in choosing the finest recreational physical activities for you.

When swallowing and oral communication are problematic, a speech therapist can help.

Short-term relief for stiffness and stiff muscles can be obtained from a massage therapist. To see if such services are covered by your health plan, check it.

A dietician can assist you if you need assistance with your nutrition. He or she can assist you in creating a healthy diet plan and ways to make meals that work with any dietary restrictions you may have.

Because they do more than just dispense prescriptions, pharmacists can play a significant role in your healthcare team. They can provide you with medication-related advice, monitor drug interactions that might be hazardous, and recommend dietary supplements and over-the-counter medicines. Use just one pharmacy, ideally one with a computerized system for keeping track of all the medications you're taking, for the greatest outcomes. Choose a pharmacist as well who will take the time to thoroughly explain your drugs and respond to your queries.

## Choosing the Best Physician

Making the correct medical team decisions for your doctor and other team members is the first step in taking an active part in your health care. It's crucial that you and your medical team form a unique bond when you have a chronic illness like Parkinson's disease (PD). To be able to communicate openly and honestly with your doctor and the other members of the healthcare team, you must have the proper "fit." You must have complete confidence that the guidance provided by your healthcare providers is for your best interests only.

Where can you locate the correct medical professional and other professionals who can treat your condition? You can ask friends, family, coworkers, and acquaintances for recommendations unless your insurance provider has very severe guidelines.

Additional medical professionals including nurses and pharmacists

group therapy for people with PD

a local hospital or medical school PD Foundation office

Ask for a list of board-certified neurologists at state or local medical associations.

your insurance provider's suggested list of local PD research institutions

**A Few Words on Managed Care**

It has been a little trickier to pick the correct doctor since the advent of health maintenance organizations and the Affordable Care Act. Our method of choosing our healthcare providers has been impacted by these changes. Most plans require you to visit a primary care physician before you may be referred to a specialist, such a neurologist. Some plans only permit this kind of referral in exceptional instances. A list of the preferred providers for the plan may also be required. If you select a doctor who is not on the preferred-provider list, your insurance will probably not cover the bill unless the administrator of your plan gives it the go-ahead.

But you still have options. Seek advice from friends and colleagues who share the same insurance plan. Find a different recommended provider if the doctor you see for rest is not up to par. You are not required to visit a doctor you don't feel comfortable with just because you have a certain type of insurance.

Be forceful if your family doctor seems hesitant to send you to a specialist. Tell them you need to see a neurologist soon. As was previously indicated, confirm that your insurance policy covers the specialist.

What attributes characterize a competent medical professional? Training, experience, and reputation are unquestionably important. The doctor or specialist's demeanor is crucial for certain patients as well. You are the only one who can determine what is essential for you in your medical team. Review the list below for a moment. Make your own list after that, and use it to choose your medical staff.

**A Guide to Selecting the Best Healthcare Team**

Are you at ease with this medical professional? Is there a "fit" between his or her personality and yours?

Do you feel comfortable talking to this healthcare professional about all of your worries and emotions, including delicate or perhaps embarrassing topics like sexual or emotional issues?

Do you believe that you may ask this medical professional even "silly" questions?

Does this professional listen attentively and respond to all of your inquiries in a language you can understand?

Is he or she prepared to spend the time to explain any difficult medical terminology if you don't grasp something? Will he or she use visuals to help you understand the subject better?

Does this medical professional welcome your partner (or another patient advocate) to take an active part in your care?

In order for you to feel at ease during office visits, does he or she give you adequate time?

Does he or she appear to be interested in you and your health?

Does this person have empathy and the capacity to picture themselves in your position?

Is he/she punctual?

Has this doctor handled patients with PD before? unique instruction?

Does this healthcare professional—a doctor or a pharmacist—explain your drugs in detail, including how they work, what they're supposed to do, when and how to take them, any adverse effects to be on the lookout for, and what to do if you forget to take a dose?

During your appointments, does your doctor or other healthcare provider inform you about PD? Does he or she offer you written materials and details on books and websites that might be useful?

Does he or she want to discuss alternate or experimental treatments with you?

Does your healthcare provider go over self-help techniques like diet and exercise?

Is this physician willing to recommend the appropriate specialists as needed?

Does he or she have access in an emergency? Has he or she described what to do in an emergency?

Your health care provider is reachable by phone or email.

Does he or she immediately return your calls or respond to your emails?

## Having Conversations with Your Medical Team

A strong collaboration between you and your doctor and the rest of your healthcare team depends on effective communication. You will have a lot of inquiries both when your condition is first identified and as it worsens.

It takes two to communicate. You must be open and honest with your healthcare providers about your condition, your emotions, and your ability to adhere to your treatment plan. Inform them of the effectiveness of your treatment.

if the medication has any side effects for you.

tell us about the methods you've found to boost the efficiency of your meds or other components of your treatment plan.

inform us of any new symptoms you may have developed.

if you want to go somewhere else.

about any other issues you are having with your treatment strategy.

## Maximizing the Benefits of Your Office Visits

You'll want to make the most of each doctor's appointment. Why? Since PD develops gradually, you probably won't see your doctor every single day. Your doctor will likely conduct a physical examination and additional physical tests to monitor your progress during appointments. He or she wants to watch you walk and evaluate your manual dexterity. He or she may occasionally do lab tests to keep track of your pharmaceutical regimen. Following are some suggestions for making the most of your office visits:

Prioritize the places you go. Prior to visiting the doctor, have a plan in place. The doctor may need to change the dosage of your medicine or discuss coping mechanisms for any problematic new symptoms. Be prepared. Make a note of your worries and questions and bring them into the examination room. Be organized.

Avoid wasting time. You should be aware that your doctor sees a lot of patients. He or she only has so much time to spend with you. In many managed-care plans, this is especially true. Your time is also worthwhile. Spend no time in idle chit-chat or conversations that are unrelated.

Get your patient advocate there. To go with you to the doctor's appointment, ask a spouse, member of your immediate family, close friend, or carer. This individual could serve as your patient advocate, taking notes, helping you ask questions, providing the doctor with more information, and acting in your best interests in general. If you feel awkward or scared when speaking with the doctor or posing questions, it is extremely crucial that you have a patient advocate. If you'd like, your patient advocate may even go with you for the examination and accompany you back to the doctor's office afterward.

Make notes. Remembering everything the doctor says is challenging. While the doctor is speaking, don't be reluctant to take notes. To accomplish this for you, you could ask your patient advocate.

Be sincere. Only if your doctor is fully informed about your health, your symptoms, and your adherence to your treatment plan will they be able to provide you with the best care possible. Even though it can be uncomfortable at times, your doctor will be able to better plan your therapy if you are open and honest about issues like sexual dysfunction or your mood.

Know your facts. Read as much as you can, speak with people who have PD, and address your worries with your doctor. Ask your doctor about novel treatments for Parkinson's disease (PD) and drugs if necessary. If you want to be informed about new advancements in PD treatment and research, you might want to sign up for one of the many newsletters available.

## Why Patient Advocates Are Important

Most people would probably reply "No" when asked if they wanted or needed a patient advocate. We're not used to asking for assistance, particularly the kind of personal assistance that a patient advocate offers. Being in the exam room with someone else makes many individuals feel uncomfortable. They feel confident enough to speak for themselves.

But you can't really be your own best advocate if you're a patient. Independent decision-making can be challenging due to the nature of PD. Furthermore, it could be more difficult to behave logically and objectively when experiencing intense emotions or mood swings.

The ideal person to assist you in helping yourself and getting the greatest care is a knowledgeable spouse, family member, friend, or caregiver who is familiar with your background, requirements, and preferences.

# Chapter five

## Parkinson's disease medication therapy

You can get relief from Parkinson's disease symptoms with the correct drugs. There isn't, however, a single pharmacological therapy for PD that works for everyone. People vary greatly in their responses to medication therapy, just as they do with PD symptoms. Some people respond extremely well to a certain medicine. Others might not be able to tolerate a medication or discover that it only partially relieves their symptoms. It's critical to communicate frequently with your doctor, letting them know how you are reacting to specific medications and dosages. You can manage your PD by combining the appropriate drugs, which you can do together.

Since PD is a progressive condition, you will probably use various medications at various stages. You may learn more about PD medications in this chapter, including their advantages and possible negative effects. One or more of the weaker medications is frequently used by doctors to start a treatment. Being a compliant patient is made easier by being an informed customer.

**The Gold Standard of PD treatment is levodopa.**
A significant advancement in treating PD symptoms was the creation of the medication levodopa, also known as l-dopa, which is the preferred treatment today. The brain can't directly absorb dopamine itself because the chemical can't cross the blood-brain barrier, an intricate network of fine blood vessels and cells that filters blood before it reaches the brain. Levodopa enters the brain and is converted to dopamine, the brain chemical lacking in people with PD.

However, levodopa can cross the blood-brain barrier and subsequently be changed into dopamine by enzymes. You can live a long, active, and productive life with the aid of levodopa. It may significantly lessen memory loss, sadness, excessive salivation, tremor, bradykinesia (slowness of movement), walking difficulty, hypomimia (mask-like facial expression), muscle stiffness, and changes in skin texture. PD patients typically benefit from it in that they can write and speak more clearly, stay more alert, swallow more easily, sleep more soundly, and generally feel better overall.

**Levodopa and Other Drugs in Combination**

Levodopa is frequently taken with the medication carbidopa to prevent "breaking down" of the medicine before it reaches the brain. Additionally, carbidopa can lessen the negative effects of levodopa such nausea, vomiting, stomach pain, and cardiac issues.

The brand name for the mixture of carbidopa and levodopa is Sinemet. Sinemet CR, a slow-release version of the medication, is also available and requires fewer repeat doses. Sinemet CR, however, might be challenging for the digestive system to absorb. Sinemet is typically introduced in low dosages.

Your doctor will then gradually change the dosage until the optimal clinical response is reached. To fully benefit from carbidopa/levodopa, even once a therapeutic dose is attained, it may take two to three months.

Entacapone (Comtan) as well as carbidopa and levodopa are all components of the medication Stalevo. Entacapone functions similarly to carbidopa by inhibiting an enzyme that prevents levodopa from being absorbed by the brain. According to tests, Stalevo provides an additional nearly one and a half hours per day of symptom alleviation when compared to Sinemet.

## Carbidopa/Levodopa treatment advancements

Newer drugs and delivery technologies are now accessible as research into PD treatment methods advances. These improvements include Rytary, a brand-new levodopa/carbidopa medication, and a more recent administration method in which the medication is administered by a tiny, external pump straight into the upper belly. Let's start by talking about the brand-new oral drug Rytary.

## Rytary

Rytary, a combination of carbidopa and levodopa with a prolonged release, was given the FDA's approval in 2015. The medication aims to lessen the amount of time during the day when Parkinson's patients' symptoms are not effectively controlled, which is one of their most crucial needs.

A dosage may peak and then last for up to four or five hours with Rytary because it contains both "immediate" and "intermediate" beads. PD symptoms don't come back during "off times," when regular doses of carbidopa/levodopa "wear off."

In both the early and later stages of PD, Rytary may be beneficial. Most patients switch to the extended-release capsule without any trouble. Nephrotic syndrome, vertigo, headaches, and insomnia are possible side effects.

**Duodopa**

The medication Duodopa is a more recent type of levodopa therapy. Duodopa is a gel that is administered through a surgically placed tube into the duodenum, or upper part of the small intestine, for people with advanced Parkinson's disease (PD). This tube is connected to a tiny, electronic pump that continuously regulates the delivery of carbidopa and levodopa. The pump itself is worn on the outside; it is connected to a strap that can be slung over the shoulder or worn around the neck. The "wear-off" effect of medications administered orally is prevented by continuous dosing.

Although this infusion technique necessitates the surgical insertion of a tube into the small intestine, it is a viable alternative for patients whose symptoms may be worsening and who have not responded to oral drugs.

**How to Get the Most Out of Levodopa**

Always take your prescriptions on schedule. In order to avoid or minimize "off times," when the medicine isn't working, you must adhere to a precise regimen.

Have a dosage on hand. Always keep your dosage pack with you. You'll still be able to take your dose on time if you're delayed or caught in traffic (just make sure it's out of kids' reach).

Create a mechanism for reminders. You can set alarms, calendars, and check-off lists to remind you when to take your medication. Alarms on some dose packs can be programmed to sound at the appropriate moment. If you've missed a dosage by less than an hour, talk to your doctor about chewing your pills. You might have quicker relief.

Avoid attempting to catch up on missed doses. Don't take a double dose if you missed a dose by a few hours. It will simply make side effects worse. Return to your schedule after taking your usual medication.

Take Sinemet 60 minutes before or after meals for optimal absorption. Levodopa cannot reach the brain in its fullest amount when there is food in the stomach since this delays absorption.

**Potential Drug-Food Interactions**

An instance of an amino acid is levodopa. Only a certain quantity of amino acids may be transported into your bloodstream at once. Your blood will circulate with more amino acids when you consume more protein, which will prevent levodopa from being absorbed.

According to some experts, consuming too much protein in your diet may be the cause or aggravation of the "wearing-off" and "on-off" effects of PD medication. However, as protein is a necessary nutrient, you should watch how much of it you consume. As previously noted, you should also wait at least an hour between taking your dose and eating any protein.

Discuss your diet with your doctor. People receiving levodopa have specialized low-protein diets created for them. The amount of the medication that reaches the brain will also be reduced by anything that prevents it from reaching the bloodstream.

Additionally, think about speaking with a nutritionist who has experience working with PD patients. He or she can assist you figure out how to eat adequate protein without compromising the effectiveness of levodopa.

Finally, discuss any additional medications you are taking with your doctor. Some blood pressure medications, antipsychotics, anti-nausea drugs, and antidepressants may have an unfavorable effect on dopamine levels.

**Levodopa side effects that could occur**

the effect that wears off. The wearing-off effect is an issue for many persons receiving levodopa medication. The drug's effectiveness is reduced over time with continued use. Your symptoms might come back before your next dose, which won't likely provide relief right away because the brain requires some time to absorb the medication. Doctors strive to keep the levodopa dose as low as feasible while still controlling symptoms in order to prolong the wearing-off effect.

sporadic instances. About 30% of PD patients eventually experience "on-off" bouts. "On" periods denote the times when your Parkinson's drugs are successfully managing symptoms. During "off" periods, symptoms resurface after the effects of your medication have worn off.
During this "off" time, symptoms can reappear.

As previously indicated, a "off" attack can cause a sudden freezing episode in which you become immobile and run the risk of falling. You might not be able to move out of a chair or feel as though your feet are stuck to the ground. According to experts, this happens because the brain's dopamine receptors gradually vanish or lose their capacity to absorb the dopamine that levodopa delivers.

You can try marching instead of walking, shifting your weight from one leg to the other, or making an effort to cross an imaginary line if you experience a freezing episode while on your feet.

You might need to take another dose of your medication in specific circumstances. Your doctor may change your medication dosage to help reduce these symptoms if you let him or her know about these occurrences.

Dyskinesia. Dyskinesia—involuntary nodding, jerking, or twitching—which can be swift or gradual, mild or severe—is another issue with long-term levodopa use. When it is severe, controlling this unsettling symptom can be challenging; once again, doing so calls for persistence, wisdom, and frequently the expertise of a neurologist who can select the best combination of medications.

Nausea. If you have nausea, especially in the morning, consider taking your medication with some crackers or juice. You should take any PD drugs separately from tomato juice because it contains a substantial quantity of protein.

Other side effects are often transient, but you should let your doctor know if they persist or are concerning. Here are some additional negative effects:

Feeling weak, light-headed, or dizzy, especially when getting out of a laying or seated position
Pain, burning, or tightness: jaw, neck, arms, shoulder, knees, ankles; chest pain, discomfort, tightness; crawling, itching, numbness, prickling, "pins and needles," "tingling"; pain with urination; leg pain, stomach pain, pain in the back or side, jaw, neck, arms, shoulder, knees, and ankles.

Belching, indigestion, a burning sensation, upper abdominal pain, constipation, diarrhea, and gas are symptoms of stomach or digestive issues.

alterations in vision (blurred vision)

cramps, spasms, discomfort, stiffness, shaking, and jerking in the muscles. Entacapone must always be used with levodopa; otherwise, a negative effect may result from the combination of the two medications.)

Levodopa can also affect the results of at-home blood-sugar tests if you have diabetes. Be sure to discuss any potential distortion with your doctor if you have diabetes and conduct at-home testing.

The explanation of the several additional drug classes used to treat Parkinson's symptoms is provided in the text that follows.

The medications are listed by brand name, generic name, and class.

There is a lot of information here to keep in mind.

**Agonists of dopamine**

Dopamine agonist medications relieve the symptoms of Parkinson's disease (PD) by simulating the brain chemical's effects. Dopamine agonists that are frequently prescribed include apomorphine (Apokyn injectable), ropinirole (Requip, Requip XL), pramipexole (Mirapex), and bromocriptine (Parlodel).

Levodopa can be taken either by itself or in conjunction with dopamine agonists. They frequently permit a 5–30% reduction in levodopa dosage. Dopamine agonists may be especially helpful in the early stages of Parkinson's disease (PD) and may even be as effective as levodopa during the first one to three years of treatment, while generally being less effective than the drug. The medicine must be consumed within seven hours of taking it.

**Agonists of dopamine may:**

reduce or eliminate the wearing-off and on-off episodes, as well as other levodopa side effects.

Levodopa dosage should be decreased. soothe leg cramps during the night.

be beneficial throughout the disease's course.

assist in reducing tremors, rigidity, and sluggishness.

## Dopamine antagonists' possible negative effects

Dopamine agonist side effects are typically transient, but you should let your doctor know if they persist or are concerning. Dopamine agonists, for instance, can activate the pleasure center and promote obsessive behaviors like excessive sexuality, gambling, and shopping. If any of the following take place, your doctor may decide to lower the dosage or stop the medication:

**irrational dreams anxiety**

behavioral alterations, such as excessive gambling or strange or erratic body motions

sleepiness, unexpectedly falling asleep

nightmares

sex-related adverse effects (loss of sex urge and ability, painful or protracted penile erections, increased libido, hypersexuality)

excessive perspiration

Apomorphine is an injectable medication, so side effects may include blistering, burning, itching, lumps, numbness, pain, rash (including hives), scarring, swelling, tingling, ulceration, and warmth at the injection site. You may also experience bleeding, blistering, burning, coldness, skin discoloration (redness), a feeling of pressure, infection, and in ammation. If you experience any of these symptoms, call your doctor as soon as you can. Follow your doctor's advice on what to do in case of emergency if they are especially severe or concerning.

## Anticholinergics

Anticholinergics, which lessen tremors by inhibiting the action of the brain chemical acetylcholine, were the main medications used to treat Parkinson's disease (PD) for a long time. Additionally, anticholinergics may lessen excessive perspiration and drooling. Trihexyphenidyl HCI (Artane), biperiden (Akineton), benztropine mesylate (Cogentin), and procyclidine (Kemadrin) are anticholinergic medications that are frequently administered.

About half of people for whom anticholinergics are administered benefit, according to estimates. Some patients respond briefly, and the majority experience improvements of around 30%.
Even while the medications may be administered for mild to moderate symptoms, they are typically ineffective in advanced PD. The anticholinergic being used and the patient's reaction to the medication determine the therapeutic dosage.

**Anticholinergics' potential side effects**
Although side effects are frequently transient, you should let your doctor know if they persist or are concerning. If you encounter any of these signs,

your doctor may decide to lower your dosage or stop the medication altogether:

- eyesight that is hazy, clumsy
- uncertainty confusion
- fainting or dizziness, particularly in a hot tub or sauna
- sleepiness (extreme)
- experiencing hallucinations (seeing things that aren't there)
- higher heart rate (particularly prevalent in older people)
- irritability
- loss of memory
- nausea
- (Unusual warmth, dryness, and redness)

## Drugs that Fight Viruses

Amantadine (Symmetrel), an antiviral drug, is occasionally used to treat influenza. When this medication was utilized to treat influenza in patients who also occurred to have Parkinson's disease, its anti-Parkinson's effects were unintentionally found. The medication can be taken either by alone or in conjunction with other Parkinson's medications such levodopa or anticholinergics.

In some PD patients, amantadine has been proven to improve muscle control, lessen stiffness and shakiness, and minimize involuntary movements (dyskinesia).

Amantadine is thought to work by activating dopamine receptors in the brain.

**Amantadine side effects that could occur**

Although side effects are frequently transient, you should let your doctor know if they persist or are concerning. If any of the following take place, your doctor may decide to lower the dosage or stop the medication:

fuzzy vision

bloating or diarrhea

hallucinations

loss of memory

Changes in mood (depression, suicidal thoughts or attempts, agitation, anxiety, nervousness, or irritability)

nightmares and other issues with sleeping

If this medication stops working, it might resume its effects after being stopped for a while.

## Inhibitors of Enzymes

The molecules known as enzymes speed up chemical reactions that change one substance into another. You presumably come into contact with goods containing enzymes on a daily basis, such as detergents that remove blood or fat stains or meat tenderizers that break down proteins.

Inhibitors of enzymes reduce or stop enzyme activity. Enzyme inhibitors prevent your Parkinson's disease (PD) medications from "breaking down" before they reach the brain or from breaking down too quickly once they do.

The two primary types of enzyme inhibitors are monoamine oxidase type B (MAOB) inhibitors and catechol-O-methyltransferase (COMT) inhibitors.

**Inhibitors of MAO-B**

Inhibitors of monoamine oxidase type B (MAOB), which "breaks down" dopamine in the brain, function by preventing MAOB from doing its job. The objective is to delay the breakdown of dopamine by MAOB as long as possible at its brain receptors. Selegiline (Eldepryl, Deprenyl), selegiline hydrochloride (Zydis selegiline), and rasagiline (Azilect) are MAOB inhibitors that are given for Parkinson's disease.

Selegiline. In any stage of PD, selegiline, which is marketed under the brand names Eldepryl and Deprenyl, may be utilized. Selegiline, if used early in the disease, may lessen symptoms and postpone the need for levodopa for a number of months. Levodopa and the medication may be combined to improve motor performance and lengthen "on" time.

Although this has not been verified, some researchers hypothesize that selegiline may really halt the progression of Parkinson's disease (PD) by defending brain neurons. According to the American Academy of Neurology's (AAN) and the Movement Disorder Society's (MDS) evidence-based standards, there is insufficient proof that the medication helps Parkinson's disease (PD) patients' brains from damage.

Rasagiline. Similar to selegiline, rasagiline, marketed as Azilect, stops the enzyme MAOB from degrading dopamine, extending the time that dopamine is available at the brain's receptors. Rasagiline may be prescribed by doctors both early on, when the brain is still making dopamine, and later on, to boost levodopa's efficacy.

**Risks Associated with MAOB Inhibitors**

Nausea, insomnia, hallucinations or confusion, as well as orthostatic hypotension, which is dizziness brought on by a dip in blood pressure when you get up from a chair or bed, are possible adverse effects of these medications. MAOB inhibitors may not be a good choice for people taking some antidepressants because the combination of the two medications can raise blood pressure. Additionally, patients are advised to stay away from particular kinds of cheese, fermented meats, and fermented soy products. Tyramine, an amino acid, can have negative effects and is present in these foods.

## COMT Blockers

Levodopa is broken down by the enzyme catechol-O-methyl transferase (COMT) before it reaches the brain. When used with levodopa, COMT inhibitors stop this chemical reaction, "protecting" the levodopa until it enters the brain and undergoes dopamine conversion. Entacapone (Comtan) and tolcapone (Tasmar) are the COMT inhibitors that are typically recommended for Parkinson's disease.

Entacapone. Entacapone, marketed under the brand name Comtan, is frequently given and is thought to be the safer of the COMT inhibitors. Entacapone, levodopa, and carbidopa are all components of the combination medication Stalevo, as was previously mentioned.

Tolcapone. This medication is no longer frequently taken because of its well-established link to liver damage. It is marketed under the trade name Tasmar and used with Sinemet to ease the transition between "on and off" periods. The full benefits of tolcapone may not become apparent for several months after the medicine is prescribed.

## Risks Associated with COMT Inhibitors

Although side effects are frequently transient, you should let your doctor know if they persist or are concerning. If any of the following take place, your doctor may lower the dosage or stop the medication:

symptoms of liver impairment include dark urine, light-colored feces, persistent nausea, appetite loss, abdominal pain, feeling particularly sleepy, lethargic, exhausted, or weak, and yellowing of the skin or eyes.

agitation

chest discomfort behavioral or attitude changes (irritability)

confusion

feeling unsteady or faint after standing up from a laying or seated posture

fatigue, fever, chills, or hyperactivity

muscle pain, stiffness, trembling, and jerking

unwell throat

strange body twitching, twisting, or other movements

urinary issues (painful, frequent, or difficult urinating; bloody, hazy, or brighter yellow or orange pee)

## Rivastigmine

The medication, rivastigmine (trade name Exelon), is used to treat dementia linked to late-stage Parkinson's disease. The medicine can help to restore acetylcholine levels, which delays the advancement of memory loss in this type of dementia. Acetylcholine is a brain neurotransmitter that is weak in this type of dementia.

Rivastigmine side effects are often transient, but you should let your doctor know if they persist or are concerning. Seizures and symptoms of shock (expanded pupils, erratic breathing, and a quick, weak pulse) are severe side effects and medical emergency. The following are other potential adverse effects:

constipation or diarrhea

nausea, fainting

increased sweating and salivation (mouth watering).

nausea, vomiting, tiredness, and hallucinations

stomach cramps or ache

difficulty sleeping

might need to take a number of drugs to treat the signs and symptoms of PD. You frequently need to take the exact correct dose at the exact right moment. With so many prescriptions to remember, you'll want to create a simple strategy for medication administration. Here are a few ideas:

Utilize a medicine schedule. To keep track of your prescription and over-the-counter medications, ask your doctor or pharmacist for a medication chart. or design your own diagram.

Keep prescription drugs in their original packaging. Keep all of your medications in their original packaging to avoid possibly hazardous misapplications. Make sure you can recognize each medication, though, if you decide to utilize a pill organizer.

Have extra doses on hand. Put some pills, a can of juice (other than tomato juice), and some crackers in your car, office, and other frequented locations. Alternately, carry a little bag with your medication and juice.

Remember to take your prescriptions on time. There are various methods for doing this. You should set your watch or alarm. Place the medications in a visible location. For instance, if you take your medication first thing in the morning, put it in the kitchen or bathroom near your toothbrush. Make sure to keep your prescriptions out of children's reach at all times.

Have one doctor manage all of your prescriptions. You run a higher risk of harmful drug interactions if you visit many doctors. To ensure that all of your prescriptions are taken as prescribed, ask your neurologist or primary care physician.

Keep a list of all your medications and their dosages close to hand. Take the list with you when you visit the doctor, dentist, hospital, and emergency department. The doctors you work with should all be aware of the medications you are taking.
One pharmacy only. To fill all of your prescriptions, locate a drugstore. You can have pharmacists who can simply review all the medications you are taking if you use one drugstore. Additionally, modern computerized pharmacies make it simpler for pharmacists to recognize any medications you

are taking that may interact negatively with other medications.

if you visit a medical facility. Bring all of your PD medications with you if you need to visit the ER or are admitted to the hospital. Parkinson medicine is also not administered in hospitals at the right quantities and intervals for unknown reasons. Sometimes the hospital pharmacy may not even have all of your drugs on hand.

Without first consulting your doctor, never alter your medication's dosage or stop taking it altogether. To lessen the possibility of unwanted effects, your doctor can advise that you gradually taper off a medication.

Be tolerant. A few days, weeks, or even months may pass before taking PD medications begins to reduce your symptoms. If a medication is benefiting you, your doctor may start you on a low dose and then gradually raise the amount.

Never take drugs from someone else. You can never be certain that a medicine is exactly the same. You frequently take.

Never utilize expired or dated medications. They might no longer be as effective.

Employ a pill cutter. Pill cutters are offered in pharmacies if your prescription calls for you to take only half of a pill. Put the tablets in the freezer for an hour before cutting them to prevent them from crumbling. Ask someone else to chop the pills if you are having problems. Slow-release or extended-release medications should not be cut.

### *A Word on Continually Using Drugs*

You could feel uneasy about using PD medications for the rest of your life. Some individuals who disagree with pharmacological therapy attempt to cure PD using "natural methods" such as different food plans, the use of herbs, vitamins, and mineral supplements, as well as other all-natural remedies.

There is currently no evidence to support the idea that you can manage PD symptoms "naturally," without chemical replacement therapy, any more than you can manage diabetes without taking medications to regulate your blood sugar levels.

Taking medicines is the only effective treatment for PD at the moment. Many of these treatments can relieve your symptoms, but you must wait your turn. Naturally, you want your symptoms to go away as soon as possible. With many PD medications, however, you might not see any effects for a few days, weeks, or even months. In order to ensure that a new medication is safe for you, your doctor will likely have you start with a low dose and then gradually increase it.

# Chapter six

# Surgery as Treatment for Parkinson's Disease

The first neurosurgical procedures to treat PD symptoms were carried out in the 1930s, and they were very frequent up until the 1960s, when levodopa became a medication. Surgery was still regarded as a potential alternative option for people who did not respond well to levodopa medication or who had significant tremor or gait issues. Technology and surgical techniques have advanced significantly over time.

The Federal Drug Administration (FDA) authorized deep brain stimulation for usage in the US in 1997. For properly chosen individuals, the treatment is thought to be secure and productive. For people with advanced PD, the procedure can reduce symptoms even if it is not a cure.

It's crucial to keep in mind this fundamental fact about how the brain functions: the right side of the brain controls movements on the left side of the body, while the left side of the brain controls motions on the right side. Knowing this basic information will help you comprehend how brain surgery can heal movement disorders.

## DBS (Deep Brain Stimulation)

An electrode is inserted by a neurosurgeon into the parts of the brain that control movement during deep brain stimulation (DBS) surgery. The goal is to regulate the aberrant cells that cause PD symptoms as tremor, muscle stiffness, and gait issues. DBS is a procedure that can be safely conducted on both sides of the brain, relieving symptoms on both sides of the body.

## Participating in Deep Brain Stimulation

Interestingly, deep brain stimulation does not cause any pain because the brain is not responsive to pain. In reality, the surgical treatment entails two separate surgeries that are carried out in quick succession—the first places an electrode in your brain, and the second places a neurostimulator and battery pack in your chest. During the first operation, you must be conscious and able to speak with the surgeon.

In the first step of the surgery, three areas of the brain that govern movement are punctured with a thin wire known as a lead that has four electrical connections at its tip. The precise location of where the electrodes should be put is located using sophisticated scanning equipment.

The main lead is placed in the chest, under the collarbone, and threaded from the brain via the skin to a battery-operated neurostimulator (similar to a heart pacemaker).

The battery and computer source for the electrical pulses that are sent from the lead wire to the brain are housed in the neurostimulator. Your neurosurgeon inputs the programming into the device.

**Following the Procedure**

The neurostimulator is turned on following surgery, and its electrical signals start to affect the faulty brain circuits. Following the operation, the majority of patients report reductions in tremor, stiffness, and dyskinesia (involuntary movements).

Additionally, they report reduced "off time"—periods when a medicine has worn off and does not control symptoms—and smoother responses to their medications.

DBS has been demonstrated to have other advantages, such as a higher overall sense of wellbeing, an uptick in energy, and an improvement in mood. Even though DBS can significantly reduce symptoms, it's vital to realize that the effectiveness of surgery will depend on how well levodopa works first. Depending on how complicated the job description is, DBS doesn't permit the majority of people to return to work or participate in demanding sports.

You'll initially need to go to follow-up appointments with your neurologist after your surgery so that he or she can adjust the neurostimulator settings to get rid of or lessen side effects like symptoms getting worse, tingling, and numbness; some neurologists ask their patients to come in at least monthly for the first six months. Additionally, at this period, you will need to change your medications so that they work in concert with the DBS. A programmer, which is a device that is not physically implanted in the body, will eventually be given to you. It might make you think of a remote control. You can switch the neurostimulator on and off using this programmer and make any necessary modifications. The neurostimulator device's ability to be configured and reprogrammed as symptoms alter is another advantageous aspect of DBS. Additionally, deep brain stimulation is reversible—the device may be taken out—unlike other types of brain surgery for Parkinson's disease.

The DBS battery pack will endure for a while; the most recent types' batteries last up to ten years before needing to be replaced through a small surgical procedure.

**Do You Need Deep Brain Stimulation?**

For some people, deep brain stimulation is ineffective. Levodopa/carbidopa users who experienced little to no alleviation will probably not gain anything from this procedure. If you have benefited from levodopa/carbidopa therapy but these medications are decreasing their effectiveness, you may be a suitable candidate for deep brain stimulation. You must be in a fit state of mind and body to have the surgery. The National Parkinson's Foundation states that the ideal candidates fulfill the following requirements:

**You have at least a decade's worth of PD symptoms.**

You experience symptoms that make daily activities difficult. You experience peaks and valleys.

The duration of your reaction to PD drugs has been adequate, although you have responded effectively to them.

Without any positive outcomes, you've tried a variety of PD medication combinations.

A movement disorder neurologist with experience can accurately determine whether you are a good candidate for DBS if you decide to seek it.

## Risks Associated with Deep Brain Stimulation

As was already said, DBS is regarded as a therapy method that is both safe and efficient. The National Parkinson's Foundation lists the various issues that could arise below.

## Major Risks

Death risk is very low (less than 1%).
Brain hemorrhage and stroke risk are quite low (between 2 and 3 percent).

## Reversible or Transient Complications

Mood, memory, and thought changes Seizures infection at the surgical sites in the chest, scalp, or brain (5–20%)
issues with speech or movement

Dizziness, vertigo, tingling in the face or limbs, or a jolting electrical sensation

## Other Surgical Risks

An increase in pain or edema following surgery
Very low chance of edema or an adverse reaction to materials inserted

## Devices with DBS issues

Lead migration is when the electrode departs from the ideal target site.

damage to the connected wire, disconnection, or fracture

Damage or dysfunction of the neurostimulator The brain electrode was lost.

Numerous of these issues are unpredictable and unpreventable. Even highly skilled DBS specialists occasionally misplace electrodes; in these circumstances, a second surgery may be required to correct the lead placement.

## Common Questions Regarding DBS

The National Parkinson's Foundation reports that the following inquiries about DBS are some of the most often asked:

Is DBS on one side of the brain or both sides preferable? DBS on one side of the brain may be sufficient for patients who only have symptoms on one side of their body. Leads can be put in both sides of the brain if there are symptoms on both sides of the body.

How long do DBS's advantages last? Although it differs from patient to patient, it typically lasts for many years. Some patients have had ten or more years of care. The DBS will typically continue to function if a person's symptoms are improving after using dopamine-based drugs.

Once I get DBS, will I be able to quit using my PD medications? DBS is not a replacement for medicine. However, many patients are able to reduce their total daily doses by 30 to 50% now that the DBS system is functioning successfully.

What if DBS is unsuccessful? It's possible that DBS treatment won't be effective. It's known as a "DBS failure." You should consult your doctor if your problem has not improved after six months.

ask a neurologist about a complete examination to determine whether there is a problem that can be fixed.

Do I need to refrain from any particular activities after DBS? Usually, it takes a few months before you may resume your normal daily activities at home. Direct physical contact with the implanted devices must be avoided. Do not climb or reach for anything that is higher than your head. Sports like swimming are generally safe as long as there is no physical contact with the gadget.

Can I work out after a DBS? Yes, the majority of patients can resume low-impact exercise four to six weeks after surgery. Sports with contact should be avoided. What electrical equipment should I stay away from? Microwaves, radios, and computers are among the safest household appliances.

Diathermy therapies involving intense heat must to be avoided. Additionally, you cannot undergo an MRI scan since anyone with implanted devices is at great risk from the magnets in MRI equipment. (Note: An MRI can be used to scan the brain, but there must be careful safety measures applied.)

I have a DBS, is flying safe for me? Air travel is secure, however before passing through the airport scanners, let the security guards know that you are carrying a neurostimulator.

The neurostimulator contains a little amount of metal that could trigger an alarm. Please politely remind the screeners that the detector wand should not be held over your neurostimulator for more than a few seconds because these detection devices contain magnets and could affect the operation or programming of your DBS if you are chosen for additional screening using hand-held detector devices.

How much does DBS cost, and will my health insurance cover it?
The price range for DBS surgery is $35,000 to $50,000. Procedures on both sides of the brain could cost as much as $70,000 to $100,000. Medicare and the majority of private insurance companies will cover the majority, if not all, of the costs of the procedure because DBS is FDA-approved for treating PD. The total cost will depend on the kind and scope of your health insurance.

**Pallidotomy**

Pallidotomy is a surgical operation that was formerly frequently used to treat the signs and symptoms of Parkinson's disease. However, since the advent of DBS, this 1940s-era treatment is now only occasionally used.

Pallidotomy involved introducing a probe into the brain that would kill the globus pallidus, a region of brain tissue involved in the transmission of movement-related brain signals. In addition to reducing or eliminating tremors, sluggishness, aberrant motions, stiffness, balance issues, and freezing, a successful pallidotomy also improved gait.

**Thalamotomy**

Another older treatment that is no longer frequently used is thalamotomy. DBS has taken its place in place of it. The thalamic region, a message-relay station deep inside the brain, was the subject of a thalamotomy treatment, which required inserting a probe carrying extremely cold liquid nitrogen into the targeted brain tissue. The damaged brain tissue caused the symptoms of PD to disappear or get better. Typically, it was only done on one side of the brain, relieving symptoms on just one side of the body. As previously mentioned, both sides of the brain can be safely treated with the more recent DPB.

Due to the fact that both thalamotomy and pallidotomy involve the destruction of brain tissue, neither treatment is now used. The gadget can be inserted and removed during a DBS treatment without causing any harm to the brain's structures.

# Chapter seven

# The Benefits of Exercise

One of the most crucial self-help methods for managing PD is regular exercise. When it comes to PD, the adage "use it or lose it" is unquestionably true. But that doesn't mean it's simple. Almost everyone struggles to stay in shape. Most people either completely shun exercising or attempt it once and stop. Exercise may not be very enticing if you have Parkinson's disease (PD) because of exhaustion, restricted range of motion, muscle and joint stiffness, or respiratory issues.

Exercise is crucial for motor function, according to research and the experiences of thousands of people with Parkinson's disease. Stretching and aerobic exercise are both beneficial for people with Parkinson's disease, according to a study conducted at Emory University School of Medicine in Atlanta, Georgia. For twelve weeks, study participants walked or ran for forty minutes each day, three times a week. At the conclusion of the experiment, their movement time increased by 37 percent, their motor function increased by 22%, and their cardiovascular fitness increased by more than 30%.

**The Benefits of Exercise**

Exercise won't halt Parkinson's disease, but it might make you stronger and more independent. Additionally, it might help you overcome gait issues, strengthen your muscles, and enhance your speaking and swallowing. Exercise releases endorphins, the body's natural "feel-good" chemicals; if you exercise vigorously enough to work up at least a light sweat, you may feel better emotionally and your depressive symptoms may improve. Perhaps most importantly, maintaining a regular fitness regimen may increase your sensation of control and accomplishment. You'll feel less alone if you enroll in a regimented workout class or program that enables you to interact with others on a regular basis.

Exercise can avoid the typical muscle and joint injuries linked to Parkinson's disease, according to research. Your body naturally makes hundreds of motions each day, constantly stretching your muscles and ligaments. When PD prevents automatic movement, you must deliberate each action before carrying it out, which may cause your muscles and ligaments to stiffen and your joints to lose their range of motion. Sprains are likely if you attempt to perform motions that are outside the range or capacity of your muscles and ligaments. Exercise can stall this process and shield your ligaments and muscles from harm.

**advantages of exercise**

Regular exercise could benefit you in the following ways:

enhance muscular power

balance improvement gait issues

less swallowing/speech issues

mood improvement and depression relief

lessen muscle and joint abrasions

feeling more in charge

feeling of accomplishment

feel more a part of a community and less alone

## Fitness that Is Effective for You

Regular aerobic, stretching, and strengthening activities are given top attention in the treatment programs of many PD patients. Here are some recommendations for safe and efficient exercising. (Ask your doctor before beginning any workout program.)

Begin gradually. Unaccustomed to physical exertion, muscles and joints react slowly. Start out slowly and progressively up your exercise level over time. Overextending yourself too soon can only lead to uncomfortable muscles and perhaps even injury.

Pick a workout plan that you can easily incorporate into your everyday schedule. Your fitness program should be something you can and will stick to, as well as something you like doing. This will encourage you to persevere.

Stop if it hurts. Avoid pushing yourself past your pain threshold. A little discomfort is acceptable, but pain is your body's clear signal to halt. Consult your physician, physical therapist, or both if exercise consistently results in pain.

Practice walking correctly. Take big steps, stepping on your toes to start each step and letting your heels land on the floor first as you advance. Several times every day, practice walking in circles, backwards, and sideways.
your toes up. With each step, lift your toes to avoid stumbling. Use toe liing to ease muscle spasms, "unglue" your feet and legs from a freezing episode, and to lessen the likelihood of falling.

Make a broad basis. Keep your feet about twelve inches apart when standing, walking, or turning to provide a wider base and lessen the risk of falling.

Make gradual turns. For at least fifteen minutes each day, until it becomes second nature, practice taking wide stances and modest steps when turning.

Look upward. You might be inclined to keep an eye on your feet while walking. Attempt to sit up straight and maintain a straight gaze.

Exercise quick motions. Move quickly forward, backward, to the right, and to the left for a few minutes at a time multiple times per day to help with balance. To keep your equilibrium, hold onto a counter or other item.

Conquer gravity. If getting out of a chair or bed is difficult for you, try rising swiftly to combat gravity's pull and inertia. Make sure your chair or bed has both of your feet firmly placed there. Ten to twenty times a day, practice. To make getting up from your favorite chair easier, try placing three- or four-inch safe blocks under the back legs. Some chairs have mechanisms that "propel" you out of them. Before making a purchase, find out from your neurologist whether such chairs are safe for you.

Make an arm swing. Practice swinging your arms freely while walking to relieve strain on your legs, reduce fatigue, and loosen up the shoulders and arms. The other arm should swing back as the first one moves forward. Swing your left leg forward when your right arm moves forward, and vice versa.

The list is balanced. Leaning to one side is a symptom that some people with PD experience. To equalize the burden and lessen your body's bend, try carrying hand weights or a shopping bag filled with books on the side that isn't being listed.

Think of a home fitness equipment. Exercise can be easily postponed when the weather is bad. You can maintain your routine using home workout equipment like treadmills and stationary cycles.

March to the beat. When walking steadily, especially if you're having trouble freezing, try listening to music. Additionally, listening to music while working out can be fun and engaging.

Maintain your leg strength. Make sure to incorporate some leg-strengthening exercises. You'll be able to stay active for longer and avoid falls if you have strong legs.

Build up those abs. Strong abdominal muscles are essential, particularly if you experience back pain. Make sure to incorporate "crunches," modified sit-ups, or other abdominal-strengthening exercises into your fitness program as prescribed or allowed by your doctor.

Take up yoga. This ancient practice should be very beneficial for posture, balance, relaxation, and peace since it includes a number of gentle stretching and strengthening poses. Some of the postures can be used by those who are confined to a chair or bed.

However, because some types of yoga are physically taxing, speak with the instructor before enrolling in a session.

Avoid wearing shoes with rubber or crepe soles. They may grab the floor and cause you to trip.

Develop your skills through practicing. Practice any difficult tasks—like buttoning a shirt or getting out of bed—at least 20 times a day to grow better at them.

**An explanation of expectations**

You need to have reasonable expectations. You might have exercised prior to developing PD and rapidly noticed improvements in your cardiovascular and muscle strength. With PD, it will be different.

If you notice little to no increase in your muscle strength and endurance, don't give up. Your illness is still getting worse. Simply put, your exercise regimen is aiding you in keeping up with the evolution of symptoms, particularly the more incapacitating ones. Be pleased of your accomplishments if exercising helps you retain a higher quality of life and gives you a feeling of control and mastery.

**How Much Exercise Should You Get?.**

Various exercises could be beneficial. Your decision will be influenced by your symptoms, age, physical fitness, and interests. The greatest program is one that incorporates several activities and is flexible enough to adapt as your symptoms and skills alter. You can create a program that is appropriate for you with assistance from your physician and physical therapist.

Daily chores involve workout. You perform these tasks as part of daily life, including housework, personal care, dressing, grooming, shopping, and other activities. This kind of exercise will keep you flexible even though it won't increase your aerobic endurance (heart and lung fitness).

a regimen prescribed by a doctor. To avoid muscle stiffness and the aggravation of other symptoms, as well as to regain any lost functions, your doctor may recommend certain workouts.

leisure activities. Engage in as many enjoyable activities as you can, such as hiking, golfing, dancing, bowling, swimming, and other types of exercise that you like. Your muscles and joints will stay flexible and strong with the help of recreation, which also offers social chances.

## A Model Workout Program

A effective workout regimen mixes strengthening exercises with stretches to keep the muscles and joints flexible. The exercises listed below frequently mimic yoga postures. You could find that some or all of these exercises are effective for you, but first talk to your physician, physical therapist, or both. It should take an hour to complete the procedure.

Walking. Walk as hard as you can for at least 30 minutes, either outside or on a treadmill. A quality walking shoe can be suggested by your physical therapist.

healthy breathing. Exhale while performing the "work" portion of an exercise, such as stretching or lifting a weight, during a workout. As you perform the relaxation portion of the exercise, inhale. By breathing in this way, injuries can be avoided, and the exercises become simpler.

Stretch your low back. Knees bent, lie flat on your back. Pulling your legs closer your chest, clasp your knees together. Your lower back will feel stretched. Hold for a gradual ten-count. As many times as you like, repeat this practice. It works wonders to ease a stiff back in the morning.

long stretch of the body. Stretch your entire body as far as you can while lying on your back with your arms raised over your head.

extend your shoulders. Place your hands together behind your back while standing and extend both arms. Raise your arms as high as you can while keeping them straight. Ten counts or longer if you can, hold the position. This exercise is excellent for straightening your back.

Hip turn. Lie on your back on the ground. Raise your knees so that they are slightly bent. With the upper leg pressing down on the lower leg, now cross one leg over the top of the knee on the opposite side. Hold your shoulders flat to the ground. Only let the lower leg to extend as far as it can do so comfortably. Your lower back will feel stretched. Keep holding for 20 counts. Return your legs to the ground gradually. Continue with the other leg.

Flex your neck. On the floor, lie on your back. Turn your head slowly back and forth and side to side without using a pillow. Add more repetitions as you are able after starting with a few. Do 15 to 20 rotations eventually. Then elevate your head while alternatively bringing your chin toward your chest and reversing the angle of your neck. 30 to 50 times total.

Your neck's range of motion will grow thanks to these exercises, which will also lessen stiffness.

stretch in a single leg strap. Loop a strap or towel around one foot while seated on the floor with both legs extended straight in front of you. Bend the other knee out to the side. Pull the strap toward your body while holding it with both hands. Your lower back and the back of your leg should feel stretched out. Hold for between 15 and 20 counts. On the other side, repeat.

stretchable double-leg straps. Loop a strap or towel around both feet while seated on the floor with both legs extended straight in front of you. Pull toward your body while stretching and holding for a count of 15 to 20 while holding the strap or towel in your hands.

stretch on the side. Widen your posture as you stand. Your left arm should be raised over your head with the palm facing the center of your body. Allow the weight of your lifted arm to assist you in stretching as you slowly budge your waist to the right. Your left side should feel stretched. Keep holding for a leisurely 10-count. On the other side, repeat.

waist turn. Turn your head and torso as far to the right as you can while standing with a wide stance and your hands on your hips. Hold for ten counts. Repeat on the other side after returning to the center of the twist.

Wall situps. Stand about eight inches from the wall while facing it. You should lower yourself into a squatting position by bending your legs at the knees and hips. If necessary, use the wall as support. Hold this posture while slowly counting to ten. After that, steadily push yourself up to standing. Although it could be too challenging for some, this exercise is great for strengthening the legs.

lifts of arm weights. With a dumbbell (hand weight) no heavier than eight pounds in each hand, lie on your back. Hand weights as light as two pounds are typically available in significant numbers at sporting-goods and budget retailers. Start out light and increase the weight as your upper-body strength increases.

While keeping your elbows at your sides and your hands up, hold the weights parallel to your torso. Raise your arms till they are straight up while maintaining your straight arms. Hold for a brief moment with your arms fully extended, then gradually return the weights to their initial positions. Build up to 50 lifts gradually. then start the exercise by elevating both arms till they touch, keeping them at a straight angle to your torso from your shoulders. After a brief hold, let go. Again, increase to 50 lis gradually.

Back stretch with foot-grasping. Legs outstretched in front of you, knees bent at a 45-degree angle while you sit on the floor. Extend your arms forward, bend your upper body as far forward as you can, and grab the bottoms of your shoes with both hands. Stretch toward your feet while engaging your back muscles to gradually lengthen your lower back. If at all feasible, hold for a count of 10. Work your way slowly up to holding for at least a count of 30 (stop immediately if you experience pain). It works wonders for easing knots and reducing lower back pain.

a set of weighted partial sit-ups. Lay your back flat. Hold a hand weight in each hand while bending your knees and keeping your arms at your sides. Maintaining a flat small of the back and your feet on the ground, slowly elevate your upper body off the floor and curl toward your knees. Return to the resting posture by curving slowly. Work your way up to 50 sit-ups gradually. This exercise helps avoid lower back problems by strengthening the abdominal muscles.

**Physical exercise**

PD can result in gait abnormalities, leg and arm deformities, and postural issues. Physical therapy with a customized plan may be able to manage these issues. Together with your doctor and physical therapist, you should create a plan that might involve the following:

exercises both active and passive. You can increase your range of motion, coordination, and speed of movement by performing active workouts. To help reduce muscle rigidity and stiffness, a physical therapist may perform a variety of stretches and manipulations called passive exercises.

Gait instruction. By assisting you in developing optimal foot placement, arm swing, and balance, this exercise could help you walk more comfortably.

everyday activities. You can learn strategies from a physical therapist to make routine tasks simpler. Hydrotherapy, electrical stimulation, heat, and ice. Your physical therapist might treat your problems with heat, cold, electricity, or water therapy.

## Other treatments

It's critical to keep your coordination and hand dexterity as high as possible. Crafting exercises are a component of occupational therapy. Look for safe and enjoyable things to participate in. Speech therapy can frequently be helpful if you start having speech problems. For issues like nasal monotone and vocal discomfort, speech therapists can offer exercises and strategies.

# Chapter eight

# Managing Day-to-Day

Parkinson's disease is difficult to manage because it has an impact on every aspect of your life, from making friends to working. Simple daily tasks like buttoning your shirt or getting up from a chair can become difficult.

If you want to maintain as much activity as you can while living with PD, you must learn a new way of life. This chapter provides helpful coping mechanisms and resources for securing the support you require to handle life's problems.

## Finding Assistance

Finding emotional support is crucial if you have Parkinson's disease. Support groups for persons with Parkinson's disease and their loved ones are sponsored by numerous organizations, including the National Parkinson Foundation and the Parkinson's

Disease Foundation. Patients, spouses, and caregivers are all a part of these support groups.

Many people are reluctant to attend support groups, especially those who have just received a PD diagnosis. The initial resistance usually goes away when one learns to adapt to a new way of life since they value their independence and don't want to be connected with "sick people."

A support group might be a crucial connection in your network of self-help information. You and your loved ones might benefit from it:

learn more about PD and the physical restrictions it places on people.

learn where to find adaptive equipment, home health care services, and exercise programs in your community.

enlist the help of local, qualified healthcare practitioners with PD experience.

Discuss your worries and fears in a safe setting.

build coping mechanisms for emotions like rage, remorse, and powerlessness.

keep yourself inspired to engage in self-help activities like exercise.

Improve your communication with the medical staff. discover the most recent advancements in PD research and therapy.

Find workable solutions to common problems.

How do you locate support networks? Start by contacting the local National Parkinson Foundation or Parkinson's Disease Foundation chapter in your area. If there isn't a local chapter in your area, get in touch with the foundation's national office and inquire about starting a support group. Additionally, you can find support groups by using the resources below:

your doctor's office locally

acquaintances or companions with Parkinson's disease (PD) or a comparable neurological condition.

The mental health association in your area

a PD research facility nearby

**Selecting a Healthy Diet**

Everyone should eat a balanced diet for optimum health, but those with a chronic illness like Parkinson's disease should pay particular attention. Numerous diet-related issues could be avoided with careful food planning done in cooperation with a nutritionist.

Just a few of the dietary problems linked to Parkinson's disease are listed below:

It may be difficult or slow to swallow.

Food transit time through the digestive system is slowed by PD. The stomach takes longer to empty. Constipation may become an issue if digestion becomes slower.

A decrease in appetite, altered sense of smell, and occasionally nausea (caused by anti-Parkinson drugs) are all symptoms of PD that may make eating less enjoyable and result in weight loss.

A poor diet (or one that is high in protein) may prevent levodopa and other anti-Parkinson's medications from being absorbed.

In general, people with PD need the same nutrients that are advised for everyone. The same guidelines for healthy eating are applicable. For those with Parkinson's disease, a few extra dietary guidelines are very beneficial.

Variety. Every day, eat a variety of foods. Include a variety of foods, such as fruits, vegetables, whole-grain breads, pasta, rice, and legumes.

Fat. Adhere to a diet low in fat. Heart disease has been related to high-fat diets. Watch out for foods high in cholesterol and saturated fat, such as fatty red meats. Reduce the quantity of fat in your diet by consuming less butter, oil, cheese, ice cream, and lean meat, fish, and skinless poultry. ingest milk low in fat. Replace higher-fat dairy products with other, lower-fat options. Complex carbs are a healthier source of calories than fats if you need to increase your calorie intake.

complex carbohydrate sources. Simple carbohydrates like sugar and baked goods made with white flour are typically not as healthy as whole grain carbohydrates like those found in bread, rolls, and pasta. Both fiber (essential for regular bowel movements) and nutrients that are high in energy can be found in complex carbs.

Fiber. Constipation may be avoided by consuming fiber, which is found in inedible plant parts. Fruits, vegetables, and whole grains are possible sources of fiber in your diet.

Water. Drink a lot of water all day long. It supports a variety of bodily functions, including digestion, nutrient absorption, blood flow, and toxin and waste elimination. In addition, water aids in drug absorption and, of course, dehydration prevention. The majority of specialists advise daily water consumption of six to eight 8-ounce glasses. Avoid delaying till you are thirsty. With age, our ability to feel thirst decreases, and anti-Parkinson medications may have a drying effect. The best approach to stay hydrated is to consume plain water rather than coffee, tea, cola, or other beverages containing caffeine or sugar.

Weight. Weekly weigh yourself. It will be more difficult for you to move around if you are overweight. If you are underweight, you may not be obtaining enough critical nutrients (discuss liquid supplements like Ensure or Boost with your doctor or nutritionist). Work with your dietician to set and maintain a goal weight that is right for you. Balance, mobility, and energy all benefit from being within a healthy weight range and BMI.

frequent small meals. Eating fewer meals throughout the day will aid in better digestion and utilization of food because PD slows down digestion.

Multivitamins. Some people can acquire all the nutrition they require from a balanced, thoughtfully designed diet. However, taking a multivitamin-mineral supplement is a smart idea in the event of chronic conditions like Parkinson's disease.

In order to combat the harm caused by free radicals, ask your doctor for a nutritional supplement recommendation. Unstable molecules called free radicals "seek out" and bond with other cellular components. Free radicals in excess can destroy healthy cells. Excess free radicals are known to be triggered by emotional stress, smoking, and poor diet.

Free radicals can form bonds with antioxidants such the vitamins C and E and selenium, which will then neutralize them. Antioxidants may or may not be used to treat PD symptoms. Research has not yet confirmed the theory that vitamins C and E may reduce the development of Parkinson's disease (PD).

To ensure that a nutritional supplement you are taking is safe to consume with your current medications, show your doctor or pharmacist the list of ingredients.

Calcium. People over fifty, who are most at risk for bone-thinning osteoporosis and concomitant bone fractures, are frequently affected by PD. You might not be getting enough calcium if you limit your protein intake by consuming less dairy products in order to increase the absorption of some anti-Parkinson medications. Don't forget to consume 1,000–1,500 milligrams of calcium per day.

The most advantageous calcium supplementation is calcium citrate, which contains both the mineral itself and the compounds that allow the body to use it, together with magnesium and vitamin D. You can get calcium supplements in a variety of ways, so ask your doctor for suggestions.

Nausea. PD and the drugs used to treat it both have the potential to make people feel queasy. Walking reduces nausea, perhaps because it facilitates the passage of food through the digestive system. It could be beneficial to have smaller meals and drink ginger tea or ginger ale. A glass of juice or a bowl of cereal with a nonprotein, nondairy creamer are also beneficial. You can brew ginger tea by steeping several peeled pieces of fresh gingerroot in hot water for an hour.

Digestion. Sit down, eat carefully, and chew everything in your mouth. Don't eat when you're moving. It may help you avoid choking and is better for digestion.

## Getting Rid of Sleep Issues

Anyone can have trouble sleeping well at night. After the age of 35, sleep issues increasingly worsen and are particularly problematic for those with Parkinson's disease. Chronic sleep issues make you feel worn out and can make PD symptoms worse. The following issues are some of the more typical sleep issues associated with PD:

Several times during the night, I'll wake up.

early morning rising with difficulty falling back to sleep

experience nightmares

drowsy throughout the day

PD-related alterations to the brain, neurological system, and muscles can lead to some sleep issues. For instance, scientists have discovered that individuals with PD have reduced levels of the brain chemical serotonin, which is essential for deep sleep. Depression, persistent tremors, midnight leg cramps, restless-leg syndrome, rigidity and the inability to turn over are all possible causes of difficulty falling asleep. Early morning awakenings might happen as the effects of drugs wear off or as a result of anxiety and despair. Levodopa side effects could include nightmares, vivid dreams, thrashing, and walking or talking while you sleep. Some PD sufferers have difficulty falling asleep at night because they nap during the day.

Sleep disruptions could be problematic for your partner or carer in addition to you. Sleep disruptions may leave you both weary and depleted of the energy you need to effectively manage PD. The advice provided below can assist you in getting a better night's sleep if your sleep issues are minor to moderate. If not, consult your doctor about safe and reliable sleep aids.

Recognize that you require less sleep. Our bodies start to sleep less as we get older. If you're used to the luxury of "sleeping in," you could find it challenging to get used to this physiological shift.

Sleep is interrupted. Don't be scared to split your sleep up into two parts: an afternoon nap and a nighttime nap.

Do not oversleep. Sleep only as much as is essential for you to wake up feeling rested. You can feel exhausted from getting too much sleep, a typical depression symptom.

Every day, go to bed and rise at the same hour. Maintaining a routine can help you control your internal clock, which in turn controls your sleep-wake cycle.

Regularly moving around. According to research, frequent moderate exercise deepens sleep while irregular exercise has no effect on sleep quality. Make sure you finish your workout at least an hour before retiring for the night.

Sleep in a peaceful area. Many people have trouble falling asleep and are easily distracted by noises. Use earplugs, a fan, or a white-noise generator to block out outside noise.

Dim the space. Even a little bit of light can ruin your sleep. For light-blocking purposes, consider utilizing thick drapes or blinds. Be careful while making the room dark if a PD patient has any vision abnormalities, such as cataracts or macular degeneration.

Cool off while you sleep. Trying to sleep in a warm room could cause sleep disturbances. Reduce the heat and open a window.

for fresh air to maintain a cozy sleeping temperature in your bedroom.

Prevent caffeine. After consuming caffeine-containing foods or beverages like coffee, tea, cola, chocolate, or other stimulants, many people find it difficult to fall asleep. Consider milk or herbal tea if you need a warm beverage before bed. Due to the presence of the sleep-inducing compound tryptophan, warm milk might be very soothing.

Drink in moderation. Some people find that a glass of wine or similar alcoholic beverage aids in falling asleep. Alcohol, however, can disrupt sleep and lead to "rebound" awakenings. If you drink, do it many hours before going to bed.

Keep drinks away after 6:00 p.m. Many people experience nighttime awakenings due to a full bladder. If this frequently occurs for you, skip the warm-milk cure and other nighttime beverages. Additionally, remember to urinate just before retiring to bed.

Consume a snack. Sleep disruptions may be caused by hunger. To quell hunger and aid in falling asleep, try crackers and cheese, toast, or warm milk with honey. You might feel more relaxed and tired after eating carbohydrates.

Give up smoking. Smoking cigarettes, pipes, and cigars is harmful to your overall health. Smoking continuously can make it difficult to sleep.

Don't overstimulate. You won't be in the mood for sleep if you're watching emotionally upsetting videos, violent TV shows or movies, or cliangers.

Sleep in your bed just. Some sleep specialists advise against utilizing your bed for activities that are better done in the living room or den, such as reading, watching television, using electronics like smart phones or I-pads, solving crossword puzzles, finishing paperwork, or doing other tasks. Your mind identifies your bed only with sleep when you get into bed.

Try using separate beds. Try different beds or bedrooms if your partner isn't refreshed in the morning but you are. PD-related

More than your own sleep, nightmares, screaming, or thrashing might disrupt your partner's sleep.

Inquire about changing your medicine. Consult your doctor if your PD symptoms keep you awake or if you need to be awake to turn over. To better regulate your symptoms at night, see a doctor to see if your prescriptions can be modified.

Follow the current. Don't go to sleep if you can help it. Until you feel drowsy, get up and engage in some other activity, such as watching TV or reading.

Attempt a sleep aid. Consider using a sleep aid your doctor has prescribed after two nights of poor sleep.

**How to Manage Speech and Swallowing Issues**

According to specialists with knowledge of PD, 60 to 90 percent of patients struggle to speak, and about half have problems swallowing. These issues could be minor or severe.

The lower face, lips, tongue, voice box, throat, and chest all have numerous nerves and muscles that are used in the intricate processes of speech and swallowing. The automatic muscle and nerve functions involved in speaking and eating may also be impacted by PD, just like the automatic muscle movements involved in walking. Additionally, annoying involuntary motions of the tongue and jaw might obstruct speaking and swallowing.

**Speech Issues**

When the muscles used for breathing and speaking become stiff and tight, it results in hypokinetic dysarthria, a condition where speech sounds weak, slurred, or out of sync. It's critical to understand that hypokinetic dysarthria has no impact on personality, memory, or intelligence.

PD-related speech issues are specific to each person, however there are a few frequent complaints. Some people with PD only experience one of these issues, while others struggle with a variety of speech issues.

voice that is breathy, gravelly, or hoarse

**diminished volume**

difficult volume adjustment

monotone (A person with PD may find it difficult or impossible to modify the pitch of their speech, which results in speaking at a single pitch, or "monotone," as it is known).

fast or slurred speech, bad pronunciation

Consult a speech therapist if you suffer from any of these speech disorders. Your results will be greater if your speech issues are identified and corrected quickly.

A qualified speech therapist will assess you, ideally a speech-language pathologist who is certified and licensed to treat speech issues. Inquire about a recommendation for a qualified speech therapist from your physician, another member of your medical team, or a local hospital.

You can enhance the functionality of the affected muscles with the aid of a speech therapist. They can suggest activities to delay or avoid future speech issues and provide you suggestions on various ways to make up for communication deficits. Keep in mind that not everyone benefits equally from speech therapy. Early intervention, drive, age, general health, and family support all play a role in producing effective outcomes.

Speech therapy may be expected to assist those with minor, subtle speech problems in regaining normal or nearly normal speech.

People with mild speech impairments typically improve their speech and discover new communication strategies. There are various methods of communication available for those with PD who are unable to talk clearly, such as using a machine or voice-output computer.

## Speech Training

In addition to the advice provided by your therapist, take into account following tips if you have speech issues:

Recognize your vocal issue and practice daily. To become aware of tiny speech changes, use a tape recorder.

Before you talk, take a deep breath to help your words come out more loudly and clearly.

To let the sound out, open your mouth. Talk in brief sentences.

Clearly pronounce each phrase, just like a radio announcer would. Make each syllable's sound more pronounced. Screaming, singing, or reading aloud are all effective voice exercises.

Practice using your face muscles to convey emotions in front of a mirror. Display your rage, joy, grief, and surprise.

Tell them you have trouble speaking, and ask them to let you know if they have any trouble hearing or understanding you.

Depending on the specific speech difficulties you are having, your speech therapist may probably give you a variety of exercises. The exercises listed below may help you loosen up your muscles and recover control over the speech-related muscles, according to national PD groups. Perform the exercises every day in front of a mirror. (Many of these activities aid people who have trouble swallowing.)

inhaling deeply. Take a few deep breaths, allowing your abdominal muscles to expand as you inhale and contract as you exhale. Before taking a breath, let out as much air as you can in one complete exhalation.

Speaking in vowels. Take a few long breaths and when you exhale, add vowel sounds like "ah," "oh," and "oo".

Autonomous speech. Learn to recite word sequences like the alphabet, the months of the year, and the days of the week. Make sure your remarks are supported by a strong breath. Pause and take more breaths if necessary.

mouth opening. Stretching your mouth as much as you can, open and close it several times.

smile that is broad. Stretching your lips as far back as you can, smile many times.

absurd syllables. Smiling broadly, saying "ma, ma, me, me" and "ma, me, mi, mo."

identical syllables. Ten repeats of "puh, puh, puh" should suffice. Slowly and evenly repeat each phrase. If you have a metronome, use it. The words should be spoken swiftly and consistently. Use "tah, tah, tah," "kuh, kuh, kuh," and finally "puh, tuh, kuh" ten times each to repeat the steps above.

Speaking out. Frequently stick your tongue out. Just let it flow from your mouth.

Gum push-ups. Push your tongue on the back of a spoon by sticking it out. a hundred times.
moving the tongue. Several times, flick your tongue from side to side.
Kiss. Several times, purse your lips as though kissing a youngster.

**Breathing Issues**

Speech issues might not even compare to dysphagia, which is a problem with swallowing. When food or liquid enters the airways, aspiration, a potentially fatal condition, can result from dysphagia. Swallowing appears to be a straightforward process, but it's actually highly intricate, requiring multiple nerves and muscles to work in unison. The brain's ability to perceive food in the mouth or throat and the muscles involved in swallowing may both be impacted by Parkinson's disease (PD).

Some people who have trouble swallowing can't feel when food or drink is going down the incorrect pipe or gets trapped in their throat. Liquid entering the air pipe can result in an infection or possibly pneumonia. Food stuck in the airway can cause a fatal choking incident. Additionally, having trouble eating might lead to poor nutrition.

**Symptoms of Swallowing Issues**

Some patients with PD experience swallowing issues but are completely unaware of it. If you notice any of the following symptoms, you may have Parkinson's disease (PD). If so, get help right once.

Coughing that causes you to become awake during or after a meal experiencing voice changes, particularly sounding moist or bubbling

taking an unusually lengthy time to finish a meal and having apparent difficulty eating

requiring drinks to wash down food due to dehydration or weight loss

observing that food or liquid sticks in the throat or is swallowed incorrectly

experiencing pneumonia symptoms and a fever

A speech therapist will assess your swallowing while you consume various foods and liquids when you visit them for a diagnosis. He or she might ask you to swallow barium before performing an X-ray examination to look at the swallowing muscles and other tissues.  will then create a custom plan just for you. Your program may include recommendations to eat during your "on" time, when your drugs are working their best and it is simpler to swallow food.

## dealing with changes in vision

Vision alterations are frequently seen by patients with PD. Some claim that their vision becomes hazy. Others struggle with reading comprehension. Another group of people complain that their "eyes are bothering" them. When a person with PD seeks stronger lenses for their glasses or contacts, the eye doctor frequently informs them that their corrected vision is perfect.

Dry eyes are another typical issue with vision. is maybe a side effect of several anti-Parkinson drugs. It is usually brought on by disease-related infrequent blinking. This issue is typically resolved with over-the-counter "artificial tears" eye drops.

Eye-muscle weariness is a complaint made by some PD patients. Double vision may result if the weariness is worse on one side. Anticholinergic medications may make these and other eye conditions worse. If you suffer eye issues, discuss any potential drug changes with your doctor.

## Using a Vehicle

If you have PD, can you drive? Driving is often associated with independence and freedom. For people who aren't prepared to deal with this change in their lives, losing that independence might result in loneliness and sadness.

You will probably still be able to drive when your condition is in its early stages and your symptoms are moderate. However, when symptoms worsen, it can become impossible to drive safely due to muscle rigidity and poor coordination. Your driving may put you, your passengers, and other motorists in danger.

Consult your doctor if you are unsure about your ability to continue driving. Learn about the public transit, taxis, and vans for elderly citizens and persons with disabilities in your area to get ready for the moment when you won't be able to drive. And don't be shy about contacting loved ones who have inquired, "How can I help?"

For individuals whose illness is under control, driving can still be enjoyable. If you believe you can still drive safely, abide by these common sense recommendations:

If you feel drowsy or unstable, don't drive.

If you've had any drink, don't operate a vehicle. Even healthy drivers may become impaired by a modest amount of alcohol. Additionally, consuming alcohol may negatively or dangerously interact with certain drugs. Discuss the use of alcohol and your prescription drugs with your doctor.

Do not drive after sunset. Even individuals in good health have trouble seeing clearly in the dark.

## Managing Sexuality-Related Issues

Both sexual desire and performance are quite personal. Some men and women lose their desire for sexual activity as they age. Sexual dysfunction, particularly having trouble getting and keeping an erection, can be an issue for some older men. Some women report a sharp decline in sexual desire after menopause. Most people get PD later in life, about the time that their sexual interest and activities begin to wane.

However, many men and women continue to be interested in and active in their sexuality far into their senior years. We are sex-based creatures.

Sexual interaction satisfies fundamental biological needs.

The need for intimacy, proximity, contact, and pleasure may also be fully satisfied in a satisfying sexual relationship. It might facilitate stress relief and interpersonal interaction.

**PD's Potential Impact on Sexual Performance**

According to research, PD has an impact on the autonomic nervous system. The condition consequently affects a person's reaction to sexual stimulation. Additionally, PD limits mobility and agility, which impairs your ability to express emotions, leads to incontinence and bowel issues, and shrieks the muscles that aren't being used. Numerous anti-Parkinson medications reduce sexual desire and impair sexual performance. Less frequently, dopaminergic Parkinson's drugs can cause hypersexuality, which can include modest to severe increases in sexual interest and desire along with vivid dreams and sleep difficulties.

Men's issues to consider. Men's alterations in sexual function may be as much a result of aging as they are of Parkinson's disease. After the age of 25, the male sex hormone testosterone starts to decline. It takes two to three times longer to get an erection at fifty than it does at 35 or 40. Most of the time, an orgasm cannot begin until the erection is fully developed. It takes longer to get an erection, and after you have an orgasm, the erection could go away rapidly. Age-related artery narrowing reduces or blocks blood supply to the penis, making erection challenging or impossible.

The brain's signal to the penis for an erection may be hindered in men with PD due to abnormalities in the autonomic nervous system. Erections can occasionally be hampered by medications used to treat PD or other health issues. Sexual function may also be impacted by issues with the bladder and bowel, notably incontinence.

A man's self-concept can be severely impacted by erection issues and other sexual issues. In some cultures, sexual prowess is a sign of manhood. It can be embarrassing for guys to not be able to get and keep an erection and "perform" sexually. Self-esteem issues are frequently caused by sexual issues.

female considerations. Most PD sufferers have already gone through or are going through menopause. This significant life shift shrinks the clitoris, reduces the vagina's natural lubrication, and thins and weakens the vaginal walls, which can make sex uncomfortable or unsatisfying. Additionally, some women go through the menopause with altered sexual drive. Some people crave more, while others have little to no desire.

Some anti-Parkinson drugs may stop working totally or work less well when progesterone and estrogen levels fluctuate in women. The issues for the majority of women start each month right before menstruation. Additionally, postmenopausal women may have hormone

fluctuations that cause comparable issues with anti-Parkinson drugs.

Orgasms might be difficult for some women to have. Autonomic nerve responses and muscle movement, both crucial for a sexual response, are hampered by PD. Orgasm can occasionally be difficult to achieve when using medications for PD and other health issues. Bowel and bladder issues can have a detrimental impact on sexual desire and performance, just like they do for men. PD may psychologically undermine a woman's sense of femininity. A woman may experience a decline in her perception of her attractiveness, desirability, and capacity as a sexual partner as the condition worsens.

## Advice for Being Sexual

You and your lover can do a lot of things to enhance your sex life.

Get control of your PD. The best treatment for PD symptoms that affect sexual function is a well-balanced medication regimen. Additionally, it's critical to use all available self-help techniques to decrease the influence of your symptoms on your sexuality, such as regular exercise, adequate rest, stress management, and a healthy diet.

Test out satin sheets. They facilitate rolling over in bed and can increase agility.

Set aside "on" times for sex. Planning sexual activity is frowned upon by some individuals who feel it eliminates the spontaneity of sex. Spontaneity is not necessary for sexual gratification, though. Planning a seduction and timing it to take place when your anti-Parkinson medications are at their best may actually heighten the sexual arousal and enjoyment.

romance again. It's possible that long-term relationships have lost the romance and passion they once had. This could be made even more challenging by PD, particularly if the condition worsens. It might be challenging for someone with Parkinson's disease to feel sexually attracted to someone. An weary carer is likely the last person to think about engaging in sexual activity. However, some couples discover that the difficulties of PD strengthen their bond. However, not everyone experiences this.

Schedule a romantic date. A candlelit meal, a single rose, soft music, and moonlit dancing can all create the atmosphere for rekindled intimacy.

Discussion on it. Regardless of age or physical condition, open communication is the foundation of a successful partnership. Ask for what you require in that area.

Get support. We all struggle with psychological concerns related to sex. When you mix these with a chronic disease, the outcome might not be what you were hoping for. Think about speaking with a mental-health therapist if your efforts to enhance your relationships with others and your sexual life are insufficient. Even the most complex problems can be resolved by couples with the help of an experienced therapist.

## Constipation and incontinence

Some Parkinson's sufferers have issues urinating. Overactive bladder is a potential symptom of PD, a neurological system condition. It follows that you can experience a need to urinate more frequently. This can disturb sleep if it happens at night. Some individuals complain that their urine flow begins slowly. Here are a few actions you can take if you have incontinence issues.

Consult a urologist for a diagnosis. It's the only way to identify the issue's root cause.

Inquire about switching meds. Bowel and bladder issues can occasionally be drug adverse effects.

Women are able to perform Kegel exercises. Inquire with your doctor about these exercises, which could enhance vaginal muscle tone, regulate the urinary outlet, and lessen urine leakage. Squeeze and release the muscles in the vaginal region while pretending to stop the urine flow to perform Kegel exercises. You can perform Kegels at any time of the day, whether you're sitting down, lying down, or driving.

Take in a lot of water. To increase overall health and regularity, consume six to eight glasses of water or juice each day (distributed throughout the day, not all at once).

**Don't drink too much at night.**

Attempt coffee with grapefruit juice. Both induce urine to assist in helping you void your bladder.

Consult your doctor about taking water tablets. Incontinence may be avoided by taking a diuretic in the morning.

Don't wait till the urge to urinate strikes. Women in particular have been instructed to "hold it" when the urge to urinate arises. Utilize whatever chance you have to urinate.

Before engaging in sexual activity, pee. It will lessen the chance of urine spilling.

Consume roughage. Eat additional fiber, such as that found in fruits, vegetables, and bran, if constipation is a problem.

Regularly moving around. Constipation is alleviated, and both physical and mental health are enhanced.

Managing Lightheadedness and Fainting

Orthostatic hypotension, or low blood pressure, affects certain patients with Parkinson's disease. You may suffer lightheadedness, fainting, exhaustion, shakiness, or a slowing of your mental processes if your blood pressure is dangerously low. When you get up from a sitting or lying down position, it is frequently the most obvious. The following advice could be useful:

Check your medication. Discuss stopping any needless medications with your doctor. Nearly every anti-Parkinson medicine has the potential adverse effect of lowering blood pressure. Additionally, discuss with your doctor any drugs that could help with low blood pressure.

ingest water. To replace body fluids, consume six glasses of water or more each day.

Put on some elastic thigh-high stockings. They can aid in preventing blood from collecting in the lower legs.

When getting up from a seated or lying down position, take care. Get up carefully and with care. The exacerbating elements definitely include fatigue and sitting for extended periods of time in a warm bath or another warm setting. When you get up in these circumstances, have someone by your side. If you start to feel faint or dizzy, sit or lay down right away.

## How to Calm Restless Legs

A motor-movement disease called restless leg syndrome (RLS) causes unsettling sensations in the legs. RLS has been compared by some to a tugging, tingling, or aching sensation in the legs. Others claim that they must extend their legs. It is unknown what exactly caused the illness.

RLS symptoms usually start when a person is inactive and get worse while they are sleeping. Your sleep may be impacted by RLS episodes in one or both legs. A person with RLS might wake up in the morning feeling exhausted even if the disorder has not fully awakened them.

Even though rubbing or moving the legs as soon as you feel the discomfort may help, it usually returns shortly after. Ask your doctor if medication could help if you have RLS. Some people find relief when taking carbidopa and levodopa together, while others say a dopamine agonist works well for them. Sometimes a long, hot bath is beneficial.

Comfortable and Safe Home Staying
More than 90% of those with PD reside at home with close family and friends. Most of us find comfort and safety at home. Nevertheless, if the necessary modifications aren't made to accommodate the

**Avoiding Falls**

The most frequent reason for accidental injuries in the home is falls. Particularly at risk are people who are ill, injured, impaired, or elderly. Since their bones have lost a lot of calcium, many older people with PD are even more at risk of suffering serious injuries from falls. Safety can be improved with a few straightforward changes around the house.

Create safe walkways. Throw rugs and loose carpets should be secured or eliminated. Eliminate elevated thresholds. Clear walkways of furniture. Ensure that all furniture with protruding corners or sharp edges is removed. Install handrails in the hallways and next to entrances. Take breakable items off the walkways.

Safeguard the stairs. Railings on stairs should be strong. Fix broken stairs, shaky handrails, and other issues that could lead to accidents. Step edges can be made more noticeable by adding colored tape stripes to the steps.

Increase the illumination. Install 75-watt and 100-watt nonglare bulbs in the hallways and above staircases. Shade your lights to reduce glare. Put nightlights in appropriate locations. Install lights that are actuated by motion and turn on when something passes a sensor.

Make the bathrooms secure. Install grab bars in the shower, bathtub, and next to the toilet. In the shower and bathtub, use rubber nonskid mats. Ensure that the toilet is at the correct height. Raised toilet seats make getting up from the toilet simpler and safer. They are sold in home-care supply stores.

**Creating enjoyable meals**

Mealtimes can be frustrating for people with PD since they eat slowly and struggle to chew and swallow. Cooking can be challenging and even dangerous when there is a lack of coordination. You can make and enjoy meals once more with the help of a few modifications.

Take as much time as you require. Recognize that cooking and eating will take more time. Give it some time. Eat slowly and completely. Reheat your food in a microwave if it becomes cold.

Have the meat sliced for you. Knife handling could be problematic. Have your meat sliced into bite-sized pieces by asking someone.

Pick utensils that are most effective for you. If using a spoon makes eating less awkward for you, do so. Special utensils with thicker handles that are simpler to grab than conventional ones are available in home-health-aid retailers.

swig using a straw. Drinking could be challenging with tremors. A flexible straw can be useful.

Pick mugs with a big handle, especially if you have trouble holding them.

Modify the texture. Consider using a food processor or blender to prepare your food. Tick stews and soups are frequently simpler to consume than other foods.

Eat more frequent, smaller meals. Less food is easier to digest in smaller amounts. You'll be able to stay energized all day long if you eat smaller, more frequent meals. Try to consume a light breakfast, a snack in the middle of the morning, a light lunch, a snack in the middle of the afternoon, a moderate supper, and a light meal later in the evening (but at least an hour before bedtime).

Use functional kitchen tools. Kitchen tools include jar openers, cutting boards with suction cups and lips to prevent food from slipping off, "reachers" to grip objects in cabinets or pick up lost objects, and pot stabilizers to prevent pots and pans from slipping off the burner may make cooking easier. Can openers powered by electricity are also useful. Using a microwave instead of a stove or conventional oven to cook could be safer and more suitable.


Making Dressing and Grooming Easier PD may affect the fine motor strength and coordination needed for dressing and grooming. You can keep your independence in these incredibly private duties with a few modifications.

Replace the laces on your shoes with Velcro strips. You might also get permanently tied elastic shoelaces and just slip your shoes on and off.

Instead of buttons, use zippers or other simple fasteners. Opening and closing clothing is made simpler by using large zipper pulls or rings. Put buttons on blouse or shirt cuffs using elastic thread so you may pass your hand through them without unbuttoning them.

Select comfortable, stretchable clothing. They're simpler to put on and take off.

widen the armholes. Coat sleeves may be too narrow for you to easily fit your arm into if you have PD. Have the armholes widened by two inches by a tailor so you can put on your coat by yourself.

Try a bra with a front closure. Generally speaking, they are simpler to fasten than back-closing bras.

Use a sock donner and a shoehorn with a long handle. When you put on socks and shoes, they might prevent sprains.

Increase the heat. For many persons with PD, the less garments, the better. Increase the temperature a little so you won't need to dress in layers.

To prevent cuts from razors, shave with an electric razor. If necessary, electric razor holders are also offered.

Other beneficial tools audiobooks. They are a great source of entertainment, particularly for those with drowsy or blurry eyesight.

Bed slouches. You can turn over in bed and enter or exit your bed more easily by using bed pulls linked to the sides or ends of your bed frame. They are available for purchase, or you may construct your own by braiding three pieces of fabric and adding sizable wooden curtain rings as grips on the ends. They ought to be long enough for you to access them when lying down.

Trapeze. Your bed's head may be fitted with a triangular handle to make it simpler to change positions.

Urinals. They can eliminate late-night trips to the bathroom if kept close by.

Wedge pillows. These might facilitate getting out of bed.

railings for the bed. Bed rails can be fixed to your bed frame or mounted on the wall next to your bed to help you turn over and get out of bed.

Improve the usability of the restroom. On a rope, apply soap.

easily keeps soap within reach. When showering, use a brush or sponge with a long handle. Replace the handles on the tub faucets with single-arm control levers instead. You can sit down while taking a bath if you use a tub chair or shower chair. You can utilize a handheld shower hose while seated in the shower if you'd like. These gadgets typically feature a variety of settings that control the water pressure and pattern.

PD may make travel more challenging, but it is not impossible. Don't stop traveling if you enjoy it. Travel may still be a part of your life with a little assistance. You'll discover that with careful preparation, you may still travel in complete comfort.

Go somewhere with a friend. Your vacation will become easier and, in many circumstances, more enjoyable as a result.

Request assistance. Being as independent as you can is important, but it's also crucial to ask for assistance when you need it and to be clear about what kind of support you need. People working in the tourism and hospitality sectors are used to helping consumers. If you need to change planes, you can make arrangements in advance to pre-board the aircraft before the other passengers and to be assisted (with a wheelchair if necessary). Your bags can be handled by bellhops at hotels and airports. Your meat can be chopped in the kitchen by the waiting staff.

Bring extra medicine. Copy your medications, if necessary. Don't check these items in your luggage; bring them with you instead.

Wear an alert-medical bracelet. In an emergency, it will provide vital information to medical personnel.

# Chapter 9

# Assisting Caregivers in the Parkinson's Disease Journey

When someone you care about is affected by Parkinson's disease (PD), the entire family is impacted, especially the carers. Caregiving is a tough job that can be detrimental to one's emotional, spiritual, and physical health. Even for the most strong and committed people, providing care can be a source of irritation, loneliness, isolation, and insurmountable obstacles, despite the fact that it is a meaningful expression of love. The unsung heroes in the fight against PD, carers, are the focus of this chapter.

The ideal form of caregiving is a collaborative effort. A health crisis like Parkinson's disease (PD) can deepen the ties and intimacy between a marriage, even though one person may contribute more. Caregiving can, at its worst, lead to bitterness and hostility between the caregiver and the patient. Both people can feel overburdened but be reluctant to ask for outside help. The relationship may become increasingly strained as responsibilities on the caregiver rise and roles change.

Managing Emotional Difficulties

When you learn that a partner or loved one has PD, you must adjust to a new way of life that is both unknown and certain. It's typical to feel guilty for having a flurry of emotions, such as rage, sadness, hopelessness, and contempt.

Here are some instances of carers expressing various emotions:

1. "I sometimes feel trapped," anger said. I have issues with my sentiments of guilt and rage.
2. Sadness: "I lost a healthy partner to a debilitating, chronic illness. There was so much to anticipate.

3. Loneliness: "Everyone is curious about how he is feeling. Nobody even inquires about me.

4. Shame: "I sometimes feel ashamed of my feelings."

5. "I didn't ask for this burden," resentment. Why me?"

Hopelessness: "Everything changes, and you realize that your lives will never be the same again."

7. "We don't communicate properly," "We've lost our intimacy. We have less closeness. How can I communicate that I'm anxious and depressed?

Your needs and emotions frequently take a second seat when caring for a person with PD. However, there are strategies for handling these emotional difficulties:

1. "Give Yourself Permission": Accept your emotions without passing judgment; they are simply feelings and neither good nor negative.

2. "Release Emotions": Find healthy ways to express challenging emotions, such as working out,

speaking with encouraging friends and family, journaling, meditation, and stress-reduction methods.

3. "Channel Anger": If you're upset or angry, think of positive strategies to deal with these emotions. Create a caregiver support group, use social services, or generate money for Parkinson's disease research.

4. Seek Depression Treatment: The stress and losses of providing care for a person with PD can result in depression. Don't be reluctant to look for expert assistance.

5. **Talk About Your Feelings:** Discuss your feelings with your physician, a close friend, a family member, or other PD support group participants.

6. Redirect Anger: Direct your anger toward the disease itself rather than at yourself or your partner. Recognize that you are not to blame.

7. **Recognize the Rewards:** Keep in mind that providing care also engenders sentiments of success, pride, joy, love, and dedication.

8. **Self-Care**: Find interests-based activities to spend your time while letting your partner pursue their own pursuits.

9. Educate Yourself on Relaxation Techniques: Biofeedback, progressive relaxation, meditation, and progressive muscle relaxation can all help you de-stress.

10. Positive Self-Talk: Swap out negative thoughts with ones that bolster your strength and fortitude.

Join a support group to meet other carers who can understand your situation and offer helpful advice.

12. "Embrace Humor": To relieve stress, look for humorous moments in trying circumstances.

13. "Take Time for Yourself": Give self-care top priority and enlist the help of family and friends to get a break from caregiving responsibilities.

14. **Mobilize Support:** Don't be afraid to approach friends and family for help, and think about employing qualified in-home carers or making use of daycare facilities.

15. "Adjust Expectations": Recognize that life won't go back to normal and that it's acceptable to

delegate or do away with some chores to relieve stress.

Dealing with a Spiritual Crisis

Many caregivers find strength in their spirituality as they deal with the difficulties of PD. Nevertheless, providing care can occasionally lead to a spiritual crisis for both the caregiver and the person receiving care. When a chronic illness first appears, people may wonder "Why me?" or believe that a higher force has abandoned them.

If you notice a decline in your spirituality, think about asking for advice from a reliable source like your pastor, rabbi, or counselor. Here are some ideas for dealing with spiritual difficulties:

1. Recognize Lack of Control: Recognize that there are things in life over which you have no control and concentrate on those.

2. **Appreciate Small Wonders:** Take the time to appreciate the beauty that surrounds us every day, such as sunsets, blooming flowers, or children's laughing.

3. Gratitude notebook: Keep a gratitude notebook by listing five things each day for which you are grateful.

4. "Reconnect Spiritually": Set aside time each day for prayer, meditation, or other forms of communication with your higher self.

5. Nature Connection: Get outside and experience the wonders of life.

Change your viewpoint on providing care by:

Consider providing care as a chance for personal development and learning rather than a burden.

**Self-empowerment:**

Use positive affirmations to strengthen your abilities as you see yourself successfully handling the obstacles you are facing.

Taking on Physical Difficulties

The physical toll of caring for a person with PD can be severe. Many of the responsibilities that your loved one used to carry out may end up falling to you. Physical exertion may be necessary, particularly when managing sleep disorders, mobility problems, and drug schedules. For caregivers to overcome these physical obstacles, self-care must come first:

1. Stress management: Laughter, exercise, and relaxation methods can all be used to reduce stress.
2. **Regular Exercise**: Exercise frequently to maintain strength and reduce strain.
3. Avoid Drinking Too Much Alcohol: Alcohol is a depressive and is not a healthy coping method.

4. Balanced Diet: Reduce intake of fat, caffeine, alcohol, refined sugar, and salt while maintaining a balanced diet that includes whole grains, fruits, vegetables, and appropriate water.

5. Get adequate Sleep: Get adequate sleep to prevent fatigue and depression.

6. **Proper Lifting Techniques**: **To retain your loved one's dignity and avoid injury, learn the proper lifting techniques.

7. **Ask for Help When Needed:** Don't be afraid to request help when you require it.

Getting Assistance

The obligations placed on caretakers grow as PD worsens. Many carers try to handle everything on their own, but even the most committed caretakers may come to a point where they need help. enlist the aid of numerous sources:

1. "Friends and Family": Be clear in your requirements communication and think about

planning a time for family or friends to offer help or take your loved one on outings.

2. Places of Worship: Religious groups frequently provide helpful support, from prayer groups to meal assistance and adult day care services.

3. Use social-service organizations like Meals on Wheels to provide meals to reduce the load of cooking.

www.ingramcontent.com/pod-product-compliance
Lightning Source LLC
Chambersburg PA
CBHW050805260726
48660CB00004B/1268